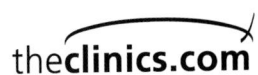

CLINICS IN OCCUPATIONAL AND ENVIRONMENTAL MEDICINE

Exposure to Airborne Particles:
Health Effects and Mechanisms

GUEST EDITORS
Mark W. Frampton, MD
Mark J. Utell, MD

Volume 5 • Number 4

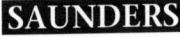

An Imprint of Elsevier, Inc.
PHILADELPHIA   LONDON   TORONTO   MONTREAL   SYDNEY   TOKYO

W.B. SAUNDERS COMPANY
A Division of Elsevier Inc.

Elsevier Inc., 1600 John F. Kennedy Blvd., Suite 1800, Philadelphia, PA 19103-2899

http://www.occmed.theclinics.com

CLINICS IN OCCUPATIONAL AND	**Volume 5, Number 4**
ENVIRONMENTAL MEDICINE	**ISSN 1526-0046**
Editor: Catherine Bewick	**ISBN 1-4160-4744-1**

Clinics in Occupational and Environmental Medicine (ISSN 1526-0046) is published quarterly in February, May, August, and November by Elsevier Inc., 360 Park Avenue South, New York, NY, 10010. Business and editorial offices: 1600 John F. Kennedy Blvd., Suite 1800, Philadelphia, PA 19103-2899. Customer Service Office: 6277 Sea Harbor Drive, Orlando, FL 32887-4800. Subscription prices are $120.00 per year for US individuals, $166.00 per year for US institutions, $60.00 per year for US students and residents, $135.00 per year for Canadian individuals, $204.00 per year for Canadian institutions, $155.00 per year for international individuals, $204.00 per year for international institutions and $78.00 per year for Canadian and foreign students/residents. Foreign air speed delivery is included in all *Clinics* subscription prices. All prices are subject to change without notice. **Customer Service: 1-800-654-2452 (US). From outside of the US, call 1-407-345-4000. E-mail: hhspcs@wbsaunders.com. POSTMASTER:** Send address changes to *Clinics in Occupational and Environmental Medicine*, Elsevier Periodicals Customer Service, 6277 Sea Harbor Drive, Orlando, FL 32887-4800.

Clinics in Occupational and Environmental Medicine is indexed in *Index Medicus*

Printed in the United States of America.

GUEST EDITORS

MARK W. FRAMPTON, MD, Professor of Medicine and Environmental Medicine, Division of Pulmonary and Critical Care Medicine, University of Rochester Medical Center, Rochester, New York

MARK J. UTELL, MD, Professor of Medicine and Environmental Medicine, Division of Pulmonary and Critical Care Medicine, University of Rochester School of Medicine and Dentistry, Rochester, New York

CONTRIBUTORS

WILLIAM S. BECKETT, MD, MPH, Professor, Environmental Medicine and Medicine, University of Rochester School of Medicine and Dentistry, Rochester, New York

ALISON ELDER, PhD, Research Assistant Professor, Department of Environmental Medicine, University of Rochester, Rochester, New York

MARK W. FRAMPTON, MD, Professor of Medicine and Environmental Medicine, Division of Pulmonary and Critical Care Medicine, University of Rochester Medical Center, Rochester, New York

JOHN J. GODLESKI, MD, Associate Professor of Pathology, Department of Environmental Health, Harvard School of Public Health, Boston, Massachusetts

PHILIP K. HOPKE, PhD, Bayard D. Clarkson Distinguished Professor and Director, Center for Air Resources Engineering and Science, Clarkson University, Potsdam, New York

MARC F. HOYLAERTS, PhD, K.U. Leuven, Center for Molecular and Vascular Biology, Leuven, Belgium

MICHAEL KOVOCHICH, BS, Division of Clinical Immunology and Allergy, Department of Medicine, University of California Los Angeles; and Southern California Particle Center, Los Angeles, California

ANDRE NEL, MD, PhD, Division of Clinical Immunology and Allergy, Department of Medicine, University of California Los Angeles; and Southern California Particle Center, Los Angeles, California

BENOIT NEMERY, MD, PhD, K.U. Leuven, Laboratory of Pneumology (Unit of Lung Toxicology), Leuven, Belgium

ABDERRAHIM NEMMAR, DVM, PhD, K.U. Leuven, Laboratory of Pneumology (Unit of Lung Toxicology), Leuven, Belgium; Department of Physiology, Sultan Qaboos University, College of Medicine, Al-khod, Sultanate of Oman

GÜNTER OBERDÖRSTER, DVM, PhD, Professor of Environmental Medicine, Director of Pulmonary Toxicology, Department of Environmental Medicine, University of Rochester, Rochester, New York

MICHAEL J. OLDHAM, PhD, Assistant Researcher, Community and Environmental Medicine, School of Medicine, University of California; and Director, Air Pollution Health Effects Laboratory, University of California, Irvine, California

ROBERT F. PHALEN, PhD, Professor of Community and Environmental Medicine, School of Medicine, University of California; Director, Air Pollution Health Effects Laboratory, University of California; and Professor, Center for Occupational and Environmental Health, University of California, Irvine, California

ALAN ROSSNER, PhD, Assistant Professor and Director, Environmental Health Science Program, Department of Biology, Clarkson University; Center for Air Resources Engineering and Science, Clarkson University, Potsdam, New York

JOEL SCHWARTZ, PhD, Professor of Environmental Epidemiology and Director, Harvard Center for Risk Analysis, Department of Environmental Health, Harvard School of Public Health, Boston, Massachusetts

MARK J. UTELL, MD, Professor, Medicine and Environmental Medicine and Director, Pulmonary and Critical Care Division, University of Rochester School of Medicine and Dentistry, Rochester, New York

TINA XIA, MD, PhD, Division of Clinical Immunology and Allergy, Department of Medicine, University of California Los Angeles; and Southern California Particle Center, Los Angeles, California

CONTENTS

Exposure to Airborne Particulate Matter in the Ambient, Indoor, and Occupational Environments

747

Philip K. Hopke and Alan Rossner

Exposure to airborne particulate matter results in various adverse health effects. Unlike other pollutants, such as ozone, sulfur dioxide, carbon monoxide, and oxides of nitrogen, for which there is significant exposure, particulate matter exposure is much more complex because it is not a single chemical species or even a limited number of chemical species. Particulate matter includes various chemical species in particles having a wide range of diameters and shapes that have widely varying toxicities. People are exposed to particles in the ambient environment, in indoor spaces, and in the occupational environment. This article reviews the information available on the concentrations of particulate matter and its composition in these general environmental categories.

Aerosol Dosimetry Considerations

773

Robert F. Phalen and Michael J. Oldham

The concept of dose is fundamental to the discipline of toxicology. For inhaled particles, dose considerations include the sequential processes of inhalation, particle deposition, and particle clearance. Several important parameters modify each of these processes, including environmental, anatomic, and physiologic factors. When such factors are considered, it is possible to identify subpopulations and individuals who are likely to receive particle doses that greatly exceed those for the average population. Higher than average doses can be expected for people who are young, have certain acute or chronic lung diseases, are engaged in exercise, or are exposed in close proximity to sources of air pollutants. Although considerable research has improved the understanding of inhaled particle doses, much is still to be learned before high-risk groups and individuals can be protected properly.

Translocation and Effects of Ultrafine Particles Outside of the Lung
Alison Elder and Günter Oberdörster

Ultrafine, or nano-, particles (<100 nm) have been associated in epidemiological, human clinical, and animal studies with adverse cardiopulmonary outcomes. Deposition of inhaled ultrafine particles in the respiratory tract is mainly governed by diffusion and is most efficient for the alveolar regions of the lung, although deposition occurs in other regions, too. The nose is also a very efficient filter for smaller ultrafine (<5 nm, diffusion) particles. Solid poorly-soluble ultrafine particles are not efficiently cleared via mucociliary or macrophage-mediated mechanisms and are, thus, likely to be taken up by epithelial cells and translocate to extrapulmonary sites (interstitium, lymph and blood circulation, neurons). These translocation processes are explored here as well as potential consequences that result from exposure of extrapulmonary organs to inhaled ultrafine particles.

Inflammation and Airborne Particles
Mark W. Frampton

Inflammation provides a potential mechanistic link between inhalation of particles and the diverse health effects found in epidemiologic studies. Considerable uncertainty remains as to the importance of inflammation in mediating these effects and where that inflammation is occurring: lung, vascular endothelium, or distant organs, including the heart. This article briefly reviews the role of inflammation in pulmonary and cardiovascular disease and explores the evidence that the health effects of PM exposure are mediated, at least in part, by inflammation.

The Role of Reactive Oxygen Species and Oxidative Stress in Mediating Particulate Matter Injury
Tian Xia, Michael Kovochich, and Andre Nel

Numerous reports link oxidative stress to particulate matter (PM)-induced adverse health effects. Increasing evidence is being collected that reactive oxygen species and oxidative stress are involved in PM-mediated injury. The physical characteristics and the chemical composition of PM play a key role in reactive oxygen species generation in vitro and in vivo. According to the hierarchical oxidative stress hypothesis, antioxidant phase II enzymes protect against PM-induced inflammation and cytotoxicity. This concept is useful in understanding PM-induced disease models, susceptibility, and biomarker development to assess exposures outcomes and is useful for developing therapeutic intervention in PM-induced adverse health effects.

Long-Term Effects of Exposure to Particulate Air Pollution

Joel Schwartz

Considerable work has been done to elucidate the effects of polluted air, most of which has studied acute effects of particles. Studies suggest that the effects of longer term exposures are more than just the daily sum of the acute effects. Because most of the studies of acute effects have examined changes in health status occurring within days of the exposure, this article takes a broad definition of long-term exposure to include averaging times of months to years. It concludes that health effects increase as the length of exposure increases, but much of that increase occurs within the first year.

Responses of the Heart to Ambient Particle Inhalation

John J. Godleski

This article focuses on responses to ambient particles by the heart. Available data from human studies and animal studies are reviewed in an attempt to find a common understanding in the findings. The pathophysiologic mechanisms responsible for these health effects are likely to be complex, and it is highly probable that several different mechanisms work in concert. Current evidence suggests that inhaled particles exert their effects on the heart via the autonomic nervous system and via the coronary vasculature. Direct effects on the myocardium by inhaled ambient particles or their constituents require more research.

Effects of Particulate Air Pollution on Hemostasis

Abderrahim Nemmar, Marc F. Hoylaerts, and Benoit Nemery

Exposure to particulate air pollution is associated with acute and chronic cardiovascular morbidity and mortality. The mechanisms involved in these effects are not fully elucidated. Research has proved that fine particles, principally the ultrafine fraction, which are predominantly derived from combustion of fossil fuel, are the most toxic. Recent clinical and experimental studies have reported mechanistic observations linking fine and ultrafine particles to the coagulation cascade, platelet function, and subsequent development of atherosclerosis and thrombosis. These effects have been explained either by the release of soluble mediators by the lungs, which affect blood coagulation parameters, or by the direct translocation of ultrafine particles into the systemic circulation or the alteration of autonomic cardiac control. Despite recent advances, additional studies are needed to investigate the pathophysiologic mechanisms linking particulate air pollution and hemostasis.

The demonstrated effects of lower levels of ambient particles on cardiovascular and respiratory system morbidity and mortality were initially surprising in light of current concepts of occupational particle exposure and acute and chronic cardiopulmonary effects. Specifically, the exposure levels, as defined by the weight of particles per liter of breathing air, at which recognized disease occurs under workplace conditions are considerably higher than the observed levels of ambient particles associated with serious adverse health effects. The possible reasons for this difference have not been adequately addressed. To further address this question, a re-examination of workplace exposure-response relationships is needed, which may include emphasis on measuring exposures to fine and ultrafine particles rather than to total particle mass concentration alone.

RECENT ISSUES

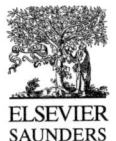
ELSEVIER
SAUNDERS

Clin Occup Environ Med
5 (4) xi–xiii

CLINICS IN
OCCUPATIONAL AND
ENVIRONMENTAL
MEDICINE

Preface

This is a good time to step back and review our understanding of the health effects of exposure to ambient particulate matter (PM) and the implications for occupational exposures to PM. That is the goal of this issue of the *Clinics in Occupational and Environmental Medicine*. Why is it a good time? There are at least four reasons.

First, it has become clear from research conducted over the past 15 years that PM exposure is a major public health issue. Worldwide, outdoor PM pollution is estimated to cause 500,000 excess deaths annually. In the United States, recent epidemiological studies suggest that chronic PM exposure increases cancer risk similar to living with a smoker, and shortens life on the order of 1 or 2 years [1].

Second, remarkable progress has been made in the science of PM health effects and their mechanisms. Many of the scientific questions about PM health effects that were originally posed in a report of the National Academy of Sciences [2] have begun to be addressed. Major research funding initiatives in the United States and elsewhere, via the National Institutes of Health, the US Environmental Protection Agency (EPA), the Health Effects Institute, and other organizations, are bearing fruit. We now know that PM exposure at levels experienced outdoors in urban environments has effects on the blood and the heart, and increases risk for pulmonary and cardiovascular events in susceptible people. These findings have revolutionized our understanding of interactions between the lungs and the heart, and of the ability of inhaled particles to deposit in the respiratory system and gain access to the circulation and even the brain.

Third, the advancing science is informing and inspiring regulatory efforts aimed at reducing health risks, a process that will have widespread impact. Of course, the regulatory process is complex, and involves costs as well as benefits. In the United States, the EPA has recently readdressed the National Ambient Air Quality Standards for PM, a process required every five years under the Clean Air Act, amended in 1990. The issues are more controversial than ever: the EPA staff, and the EPA's own Clean Air Scientific Advisory Committee (CASAC) recommended tightening of air quality standards for fine PM and the introduction of a new standard for coarse PM, based on an extensive review of the scientific evidence [1]. However, the

doi:10.1016/j.coem.2006.07.009

EPA administrator has promulgated less stringent standards for fine PM than those recommended by the CASAC, and did not recommend a coarse PM standard. Scientists knowledgeable about the issues have expressed surprise and concern at the failure of the US EPA to take its own advice [3].

Fourth, risks to workers from occupational exposures to PM are beginning to get long-overdue attention, and these risks are reviewed in this issue. Workers in "dusty" occupations are often exposed to PM concentrations that far exceed ambient urban levels, without obvious acute health consequences; this has occasionally been cited as evidence against PM-related health effects. However, recent evidence suggests that workplace PM exposure does carry long-term pulmonary and cardiovascular risks.

And what do we see in our crystal ball for the future? As in the past decade, the next should see formidable improvements in our understanding, and perhaps even control, of both individual and societal risks. The likelihood of an adverse response to an inhaled pollutant depends on the degree of exposure to the pollutant and on individual characteristics that determine the susceptibility of the exposed person. Although we have made significant progress in characterizing components of exposure, the challenges to identify factors responsible for individual susceptibility remain. Extensive use has been made of inbred mouse strains with varying susceptibility to air pollutant–induced lung injury and inflammation, particularly with ozone and PM [4]. In humans, one of the candidate genes most implicated in air pollution responses is GSTM1, an important enzyme in the glutathione pathway for protection against oxidant injury [5]. GSTM1 has a null allele with no protein expression, which confers reduction in antioxidant protection. This allele is present in 40% of the population of the United States. Children with the GSTM1 null allele have reduced lung function growth [6]. Children in Mexico City who carry the GSTM1 null appear to be more susceptible to the effects of ambient ozone exposure [7]. GSTM1 and GSTP1 polymorphisms may also play a role in enhancing the nasal IgE response to diesel exhaust particle exposure [8]. Other important susceptibility genes will surface. Furthermore, with the rapid advances in proteomics and genomics and their incorporation into the emerging discipline of molecular epidemiology, the potential for unraveling susceptibility at the population level appears as a realistic goal.

In addition, efforts to identify and link specific components of the PM mix with various PM-associated health effects are intensifying. As we better understand these relationships, the tool of source apportionment becomes increasingly important for controlling exposures. And perhaps most importantly, major sources of pollutants may be disappearing; for example, the promise of "clean" diesel lies in the immediate future. Nevertheless, the global burden of disease as a consequence of air pollution remains a growing threat [9]. Time-series epidemiological studies have shown increased risk for air pollution mortality and morbidity in groups with lower socioeconomic status. This has implications for growing urban populations, in both developed and underdeveloped countries. But as this volume of the *Clinics in Occupational and Environmental Medicine of North America* indicates, much progress has been made, and our understanding of the relationship between increased individual and population susceptibility, genes, and environment promises important benefits to society.

Mark W. Frampton, MD
Division of Pulmonary and Critical Care Medicine
University of Rochester Medical Center
601 Elmwood Avenue
Rochester, NY 14642, USA

E-mail address: mark_frampton@urmc.rochester.edu

Mark J. Utell, MD
Division of Pulmonary and Critical Care Medicine
University of Rochester School of Medicine and Dentistry
575 Elmwood Avenue
Rochester, NY 14642, USA

E-mail address: mark_utell@urmc.rochester.edu

References

[1] US Environmental Protection Agency and Clean Air Scientific Advisory Committee. Review of the national ambient air quality standards for particulate matter: policy assessment of scientific and technical information. Office of Air Quality Planning and Standards staff paper. Washington, DC: US Environmental Protection Agency; 2005.

[2] National Research Council and Committee on Research Priorities for Airborne Particulate Matter. Research priorities for airborne particulate matter: I. immediate priorities and a long-range research portfolio. Washington, DC: National Academy Press; 1998.

[3] Rom WN, Samet JM. Small particles with big effects. Am J Respir Crit Care Med 2006;173(4): 365–6.

[4] Kleeberger SR. Genetic aspects of susceptibility to air pollution. Eur Respir J 2003;40(Suppl): S52–6.

[5] Peden DB. The epidemiology and genetics of asthma risk associated with air pollution. J Allergy Clin Immunol 2005;115:213–9.

[6] Gilliland FD, Gauderman WJ, Vora H, et al. Effects of glutathione-S-transferase M1, T1, and P1 on childhood lung function growth. Am J Respir Crit Care Med 2002;166:710–6.

[7] Romieu I, Sienra-Monge JJ, Ramirez-Aguilar M, et al. Genetic polymorphism of GSTM1 and antioxidant supplementation influence lung function in relation to ozone exposure in asthmatic children in Mexico City. Thorax 2004;59:8–10.

[8] Gilliland FD, Li YF, Saxon A, et al. Effect of glutathione-S-transferase M1 and P1 genotypes on xenobiotic enhancement of allergic responses: randomised, placebo-controlled crossover study. Lancet 2004;363:119–25.

[9] O'Neill MS, Jerrett M, Kawachi I, et al. Health, wealth, and air pollution: advancing theory and methods. Environ Health Perspect 2003;111:1861–70.

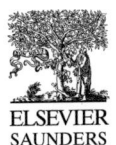

ELSEVIER
SAUNDERS

Clin Occup Environ Med
5 (4) 747–771

CLINICS IN
OCCUPATIONAL AND
ENVIRONMENTAL
MEDICINE

Exposure to Airborne Particulate Matter in the Ambient, Indoor, and Occupational Environments

Philip K. Hopke, PhD[a],*, Alan Rossner, PhD[a,b]

[a]Center for Air Resources Engineering and Science, Clarkson University,
8 Clarkson Avenue, Potsdam, NY 13699, USA
[b]Department of Biology, 157 Clarkson Science Center, Clarkson University,
PO Box 5805, Potsdam, NY 13699-5805, USA

It is clear that exposure to airborne particulate matter (PM) results in various adverse health effects. Unlike other pollutants, such as ozone, sulfur dioxide, carbon monoxide, and oxides of nitrogen, for which there is significant exposure, PM exposure is much more complex because it is not a single chemical species or even a limited number of chemical species. PM includes various chemical species in particles having a wide range of diameters and shapes that have widely varying toxicities. People are exposed to particles in the ambient environment, in indoor spaces, including homes and offices, and in the occupational environment. This article reviews the information available on the concentrations of PM and its composition in these general environmental categories.

Particulate matter characteristics

Fig. 1 provides a schematic view of PM size distributions displayed as number, surface area, and volume distributions. There are multiple peaks or modes in the size distributions. The number size distribution is dominated by the smallest size mode, the nuclei mode. Particle surface is largely in particles in the accumulation mode from 0.1 to 1.0 μm, whereas particle volume or mass, which is volume multiplied by the density, peaks in the coarse mode. These different sized particles are produced by different physical chemical processes and possess different chemical compositions.

---

* Corresponding author.
E-mail address: hopkepk@clarkson.edu (P.K. Hopke).

1526-0046/06/$ - see front matter © 2006 Elsevier Inc. All rights reserved.
doi:10.1016/j.coem.2006.08.001

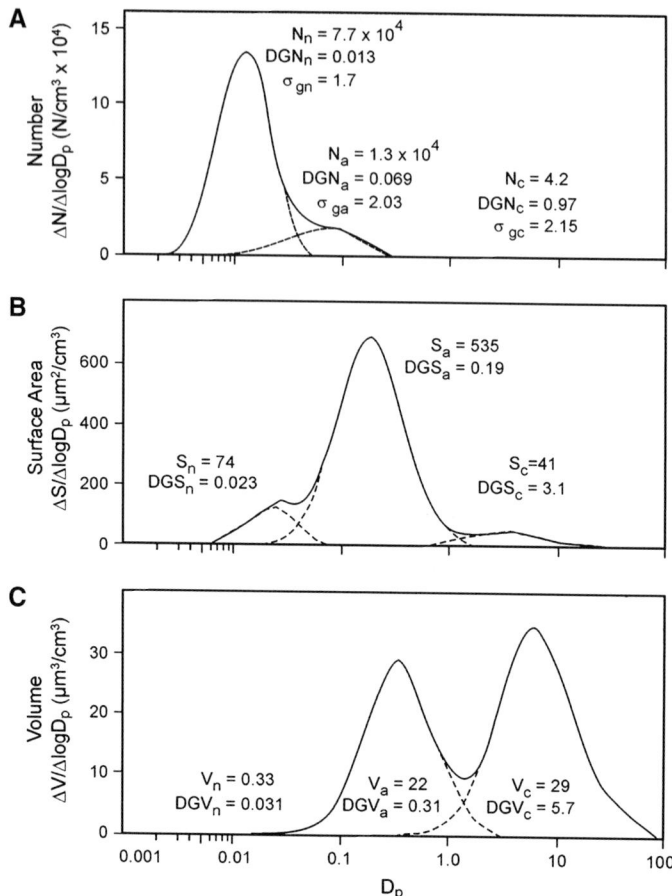

Fig. 1. Distribution of coarse (c), accumulation (a), and nuclei (n) mode particles by three characteristics: (1) number (N), (2) surface area (S), and (3) volume (V) for the grand average con-
tinental size distribution. DGV, geometric mean diameter by volume; DGS, geometric mean
diameter by surface area; DGN, geometric mean diameter by number; D_p, particle diameter.
(*From* US Environmental Protection Agency. Air quality data analysis technical support document for the proposed interstate air quality rule. Report no. EPA/600/P-99/002aF. Research
Triangle Park (NC): Office of Air Quality Planning and Standards; 2004.)

Measurements of the airborne PM concentrations generally are not done
on the basis of these physical chemical modes in the size distributions, however, but on particle size definitions based on public health policy. Fig. 2 presents the size fraction definitions commonly used by regulatory agencies for
particle monitoring. These size fractions are implemented through size selective inlets designed to aerodynamically permit penetration of particles
less than the defined size fraction. The first air quality standards in the United
States were for total suspended particles, which is a poorly defined subset of
the size distribution. PM_{10} was defined by the US Environmental Protection

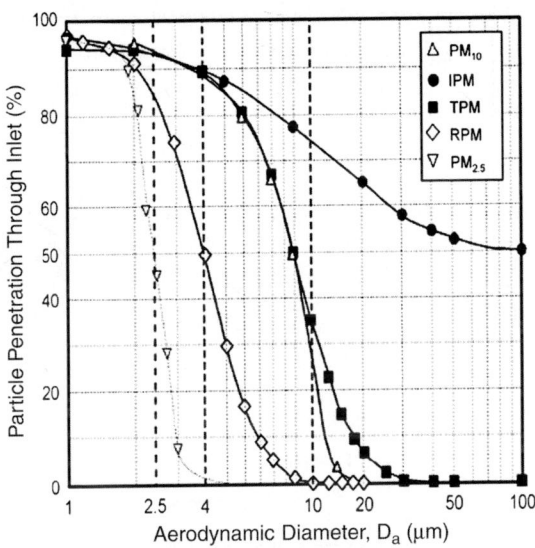

Fig. 2. Size dependence of the particle sampling definitions for US ambient air quality standards (PM_{10} and $PM_{2.5}$) and occupational exposure measures (inhalable, thoracic, and respirable particulate matter [IPM, TPM, and RPM, respectively]). (*From* Environmental Protection Agency. Air quality criteria for particulate matter. Report no. EPA/600/P-99/002aF. Research Triangle Park (NC): National Center for Environmental Assessment; 2004.)

Agency (EPA) in 1987, when it promulgated the first size-segregated particle size standard [1]. Subsequently, a $PM_{2.5}$ standard was defined in 1997 [2,3]. In the occupational exposure area, it has been more common to consider inhalable, thoracic, and respirable PM. Fig. 3 shows the results of the ambient air quality size definitions applied to the typical ambient airborne particle size distribution. Currently, the US EPA is likely to define a new ambient air quality standard for coarse particles that will be urban coarse PM with its size between $PM_{2.5}$ and PM_{10}. Because there are regulatory standards in place for $PM_{2.5}$ and PM_{10}, there are significant amounts of data for airborne PM mass concentrations. Particle monitoring networks have been deployed to provide particle composition data for urban and rural areas across the United States. Although there are not as extensive monitoring networks elsewhere in the world, there are data characterizing the mass concentrations and compositions of particles around the world. Much more limited data are available for indoor and occupational PM concentrations and compositions.

Ambient particulate matter mass concentrations

United States

Measurements of PM_{10} began in the late 1980s after the promulgation of the 1987 ambient air quality standard. Subsequently, the European Union

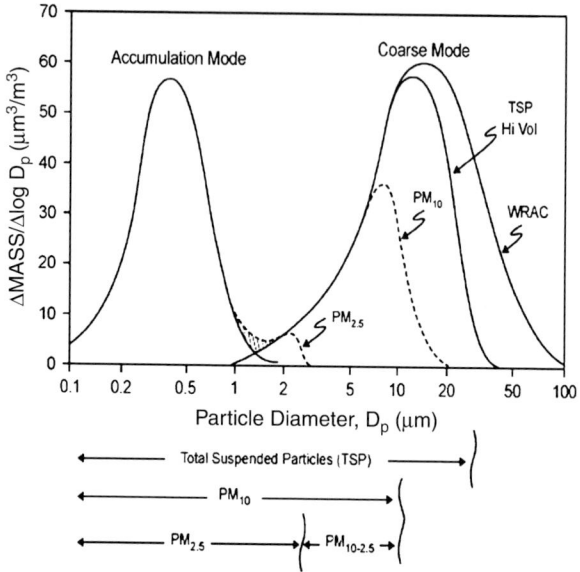

Fig. 3. Schematic view of the particle mass distribution shows the size discrimination provided by $PM_{2.5}$, PM_{10}, total suspended particulate matter (TSP), and wide-range aerosol classifier (WRAC) that collects the entire coarse mode aerosol. (*From* Lundgren DA, Burton RM. Effect of particle size distribution on the cut point between fine and coarse ambient mass fractions. In: Phalen RF, Bates DV, editors. Proceedings of the colloquium on particulate air pollution and human mortality and morbidity. Inhal Toxicol 1995;7:131–48; with permission.)

adopted a PM_{10} standard [4]. The data from the US monitoring efforts have been compiled [5]. Fig. 4 shows the mean and ninety-eighth percentile values. In general there has been a decrease in concentration across the United States so that the number of locations in nonattainment of the PM_{10} standard is limited. In general, concentrations of PM_{10} have been controlled in urban areas through aggressive control of road dust though street sweeping and related activities. Beginning in the mid-1990s, the focus of interest has shifted toward smaller sized particles ($PM_{2.5}$) based on epidemiologic studies that suggested that the smaller particles were more directly related to observed adverse health effects. In 1997, the US EPA promulgated new PM_{10} ambient air quality standards as a measure of the exposure of the public to coarse particles. A lawsuit contested the use of PM_{10} as an appropriate measure of coarse particle exposure, however, and the court agreed. The US EPA chose not to contest this finding, and a new standard based on particles in the size range from 2.5 to 10 μm is expected to be promulgated as a new national ambient air quality standard along with a $PM_{2.5}$ standard.

$PM_{2.5}$ measurements for determining compliance with the 1997 $PM_{2.5}$ ambient air quality standards began in 1999. The maps for the $PM_{2.5}$

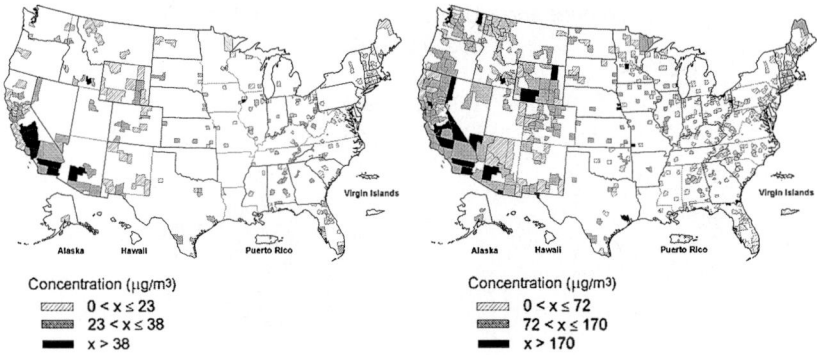

Fig. 4. Maps of 1999–2000 PM₁₀ mean (*left*) and 98ᵗʰ percentile concentrations (*right*). (*From* US Environmental Protection Agency. Aerometric information retrieval system. Research Triangle Park (NC): Office of Air Quality Planning and Standards; 2002.)

mass concentration mean and ninety-eighth percentile values are shown in Fig. 5.

In December 2004, the US EPA declared areas of nonattainment of the 1997 national ambient air quality standard for $PM_{2.5}$. Fig. 6 shows those areas that have exceeded the 15 μg/m³ annual average standard. The areas of nonattainment are concentrated around major urban areas in the eastern US and in California. Currently, the US EPA is reviewing the $PM_{2.5}$ standards and is likely to reduce the concentrations permitted for attainment of the annual average and 24-hour standards.

Europe

There are more limited European data for urban PM_{10} concentrations. The European Union only imposed air quality standards for PM_{10} in

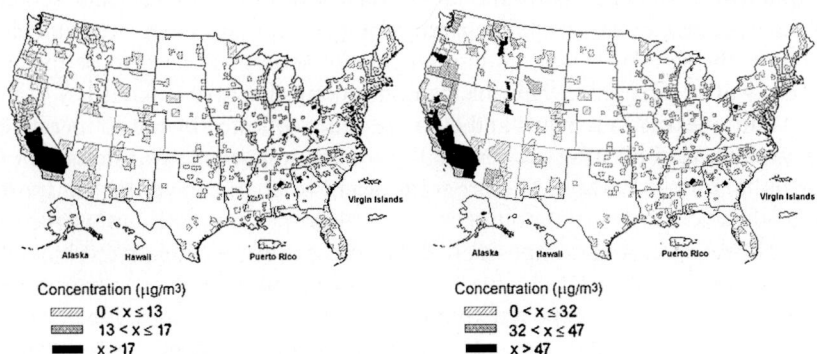

Fig. 5. Maps of 1999–2000 PM₂.₅ mean (*left*) and 98ᵗʰ percentile concentrations (*right*). (*From* US Environmental Protection Agency. Aerometric information retrieval system. Research Triangle Park (NC): Office of Air Quality Planning and Standards; 2002.)

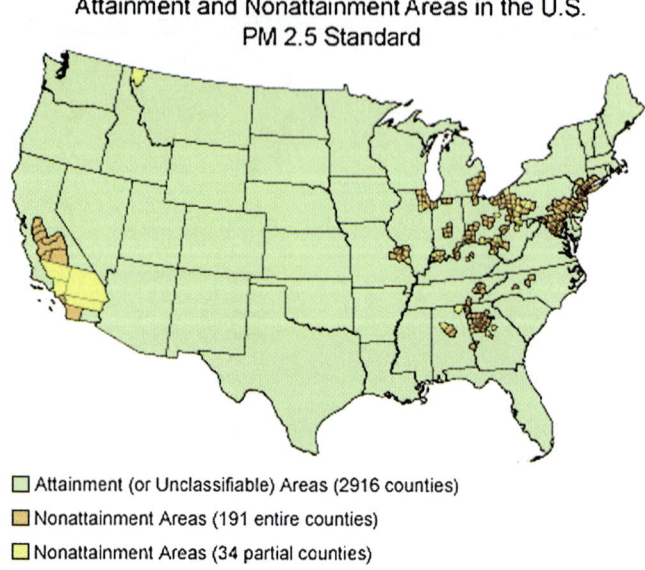

Attainment and Nonattainment Areas in the U.S.
PM 2.5 Standard

☐ Attainment (or Unclassifiable) Areas (2916 counties)
☐ Nonattainment Areas (191 entire counties)
☐ Nonattainment Areas (34 partial counties)

Fig. 6. Map of the United States shows areas in nonattainment of the $PM_{2.5}$ ambient air quality standard. (Available at: http://www.epa.gov/air/oaqps/particles/designations/documents/final/ nonattaingreen.htm. Accessed July 13, 2006.)

1999 that started to be enforced in 2005. Van Dingenen and colleagues [6] summarized PM_{10} and $PM_{2.5}$ mass concentration data across Europe. Fig. 7 shows the locations from which the data were obtained.

European Union directive 1999/30/CE set annual mean concentration standards at 40 $\mu g/m^3$ in 2005 that reduces to 20 $\mu g/m^3$ in 2010. The daily standard is 50 $\mu g/m^3$, not to be exceeded more than 35 times in 2005 and 7 times in 2010. The distributional characteristics of the PM_{10} and $PM_{2.5}$ mass concentrations are summarized in Fig. 8. Several cities are unlikely to meet the standards, and additional control action will need to be taken. There will be even greater problems in attaining the 2010 standards.

Additional measurements and data are being collected by the cooperative program for monitoring and evaluation of the long-range transmission of air pollutants in Europe. The program began to characterize the transport of acidic and heavy metal pollutants across Europe, but it currently collects particulate mass and composition data across Europe. Relatively limited time series of data are available, but a growing body of data is becoming available to assess the exposure to PM in major European cities. Fig. 9 presents a depiction of $PM_{2.5}$ concentrations measured through the European evaluation and monitoring program in 2003. The figure indicates several locations that would exceed the US national ambient air quality standard annual average standard concentration of 15 $\mu g/m^3$.

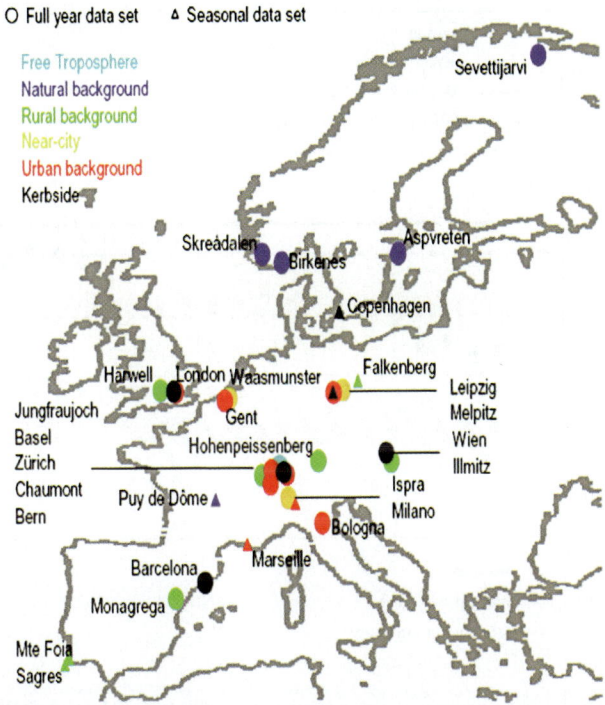

Fig. 7. Locations from which PM mass concentrations were measured and summarized. (*From* Van Dingenen R, Raes F, Putaud JP, et al. A European aerosol phenomenology. I. Physical characteristics of particulate matter at kerbside, urban, rural and background sites in Europe. Atmospheric Environ 2004;38:2561–77; with permission.)

Asia

Across Asia, there are relatively limited measurements, and in general, the measured quantity is total suspended particles. As part of its review of health effects epidemiologic studies, the Health Effects Institute [7] compared total suspended particles and gaseous pollutant concentrations in cities in several countries across Asia (Fig. 10). Although it is difficult to compare total suspended particles with PM_{10} standards because of the significant quantity of mass in sizes larger than 10 μm, concentrations tend to be high in the large cities of Asia and air quality is a major environmental problem across the region.

Some limited monitoring of $PM_{2.5}$ and PM_{10} is being conducted in major Asian cities [8] under the auspices of the International Atomic Energy Agency using a stacked filter unit sampler [9]. Fig. 11 shows the distributions of fine particles ($PM_{2.2}$) averaged over 2001 and 2002. There are high concentrations of fine PM in several locations. Most of the locations outside of Australia and New Zealand would be in violation of the US annual average standards, and many also would violate the 24-hour ninety-eighth

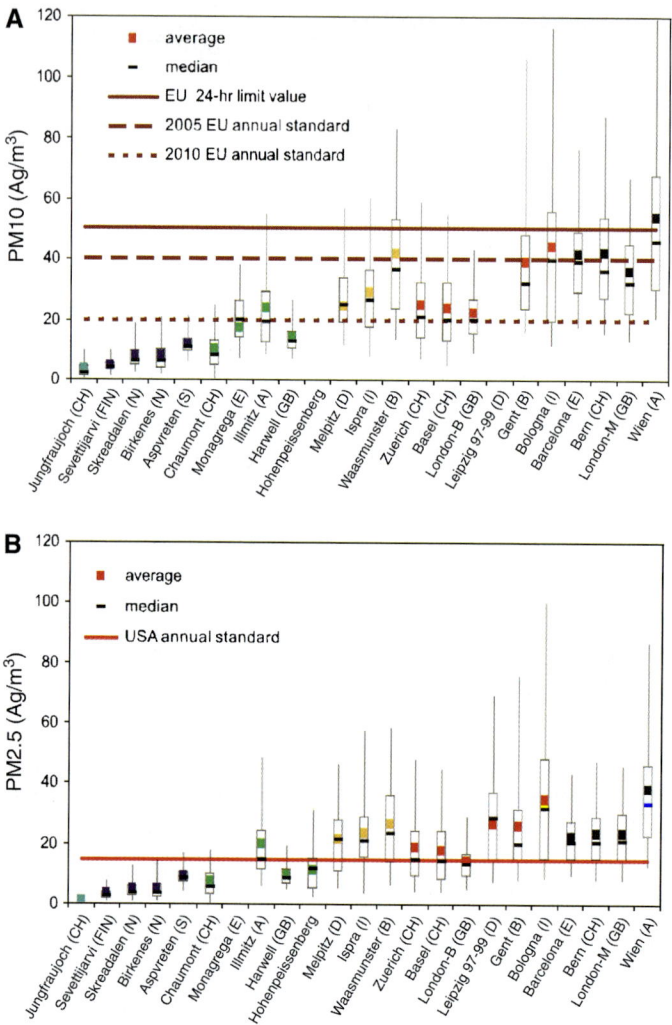

Fig. 8. Annual averages of PM$_{10}$ (*a*) and PM$_{2.5}$ (*b*) mass concentrations, including the 5%, 25%, 50% (median) 75%, and 95% of their 24-hour integrated concentrations. (*From* Van Dingenen R, Raes F, Putaud JP, et al. A European aerosol phenomenology. I. Physical characteristics of particulate matter at kerbside, urban, rural and background sites in Europe. Atmos Environ 2004;38:2561–77; with permission.)

percentile standard. These locations have various problems, including burning of biofuels for cooking and home heating, which lead to high concentrations of fine PM and black carbon. Many of these countries are finally phasing lead out of motor fuels, but the widespread use of two-stroke engines produces significant contributions to the fine PM. Bangladesh recently banned the use of two-stroke, three-wheeled "baby" taxis, which reduced the concentration of fine PM in a high traffic area of Dhaka by more

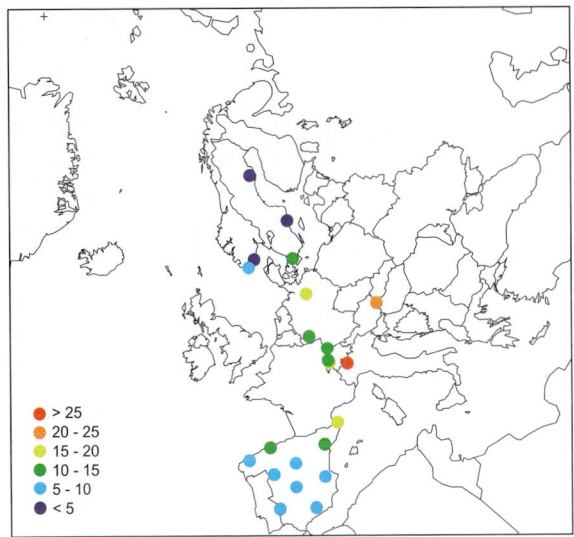

Fig. 9. Plot of $PM_{2.5}$ concentrations measured in 2003 at various European Monitoring and Evaluation Program sites in cities across Europe. (*From* Norwegian Institute for Air Research. Measurements of particulate matter: status report. Report No. EMEP/CCC-Report 5/2005. Kjeller, Norway: Norwegian Institute for Air Research; 2005.)

than 30% [10]. Extensive efforts by agencies such as the World Bank and the Asian Development Bank are starting to have an impact on the particle concentrations in several locations, but more attention is needed to address the currently high concentrations seen across the region.

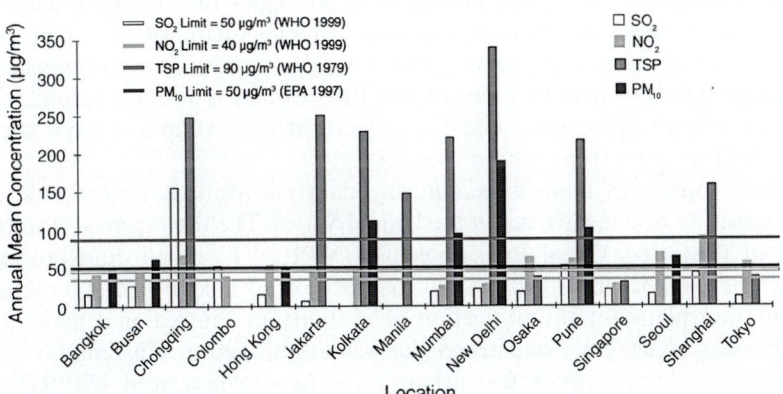

Fig. 10. Plot of pollutant concentrations in areas of Asia where epidemiologic studies have been completed. (*From* HEI International Science Advisory Committee. Health effects of outdoor air pollution in developing, countries of Asian: a literature review. Special Report 15. Boston (MA): Health Effects Institute; 2004. Reprinted with permission from the Health Effects Institute, Boston, MA.)

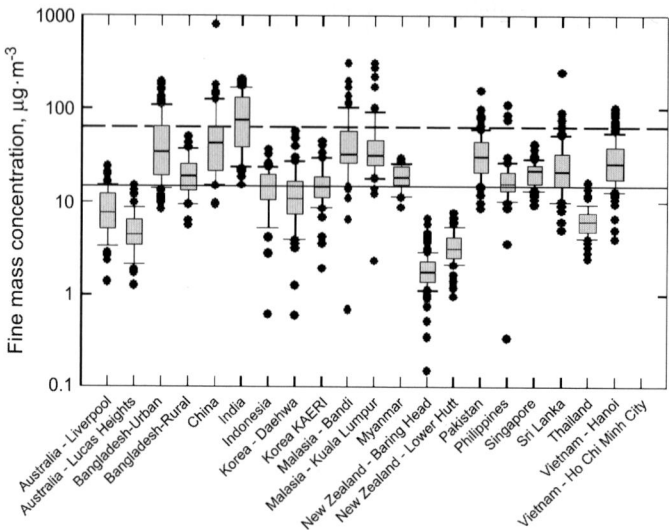

Fig. 11. Box and whisker plot shows the distributions of $PM_{2.2}$ concentrations measured in 2001 and 2002 across Asia.

Ambient particulate matter composition

With the promulgation of the new PM national ambient air quality standards ($PM_{2.5}$), the designated nonattainment areas and surrounding regions may need to reduce emission of fine particles and their precursors to permit those areas to attain the national ambient air quality standard. Development of efficient air quality management strategies requires knowledge of the sources that contribute to the problem and quantitatively apportion those contributions. Determining $PM_{2.5}$ source contributions is complicated because typically half or more of the $PM_{2.5}$ mass is formed secondarily, which obscures the origins. $PM_{2.5}$ also has a lifetime of up to 7 days, which enables transport from distant sources.

Two sources of ambient monitoring data are available to examine the composition of fine particles in the United States. The Interagency Monitoring of Protected Visual Environments (IMPROVE) monitoring program [11] was established in 1985 to aid the creation of federal and state implementation plans for the protection of visibility in 156 national parks and wilderness areas. Only one urban site was established in Washington, DC, although subsequently a few urban areas have experienced IMPROVE-protocol sampling and analyses. A long-time series of IMPROVE data is available from several sites, particularly in the western United States. As part of the enhanced monitoring that was implemented after the promulgation of $PM_{2.5}$ standards, additional IMPROVE sites were established, particularly in the eastern and midwestern United States.

To help understand levels of PM$_{2.5}$ and their chemical components in urban areas and obtain apportionments between locally generated versus transported PM, the US EPA has deployed a network of samplers to provide chemical composition data on the ambient aerosol across the United States. Beginning in 2000, the US EPA's PM$_{2.5}$ speciation trends network was implemented. These data are starting to be available over a sufficient period of time to permit their use in source apportionment [12] and provide a basis for examining the composition of urban fine PM.

These networks proved speciated PM$_{2.5}$ data using a 1-in-3 day sampling protocol. In both networks, elements, inorganic ions, and carbon (elemental and organic) are measured. Different methods are in use for some of the species, however, and there are problems regarding direct use of the data from both networks for spatial analysis of particle compositions across the country. For the results presented in this article, only the major components of PM$_{2.5}$ mass are presented. Major components include sulfate, ammonium, nitrate, total carbonaceous mass (based on organic and elemental carbon), and crustal material (which is based on the weighted average of five trace elements). Urban compositions based on speciation trends network data from 2000 to 2002 are shown in Fig. 12.

It can be seen that the eastern US is dominated by sulfate and carbon, with most of the carbon being organic carbon. There are winter/summer

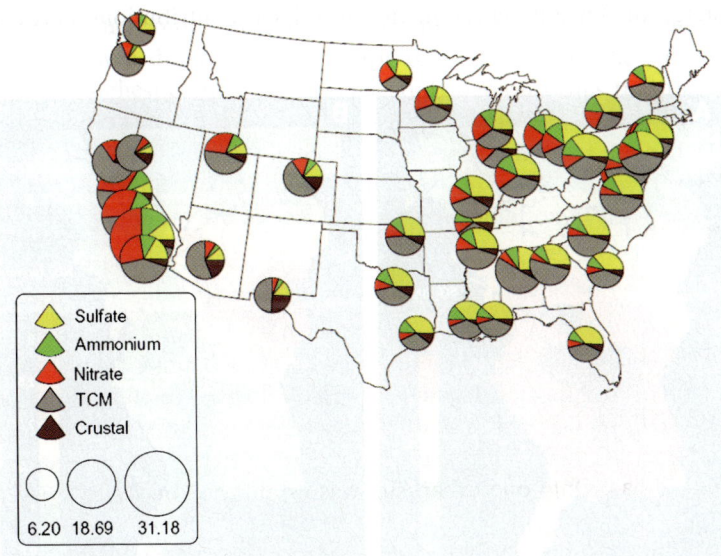

Fig. 12. Plot shows the composition of PM$_{2.5}$ in urban areas of the United States based on speciation trends network data collected through the end of 2002. (*From* US Environmental Protection Agency. Air quality data analysis technical support document for the proposed interstate air quality rule. Research Triangle Park (NC): Office of Air Quality Planning and Standards; 2004.)

"Soil" was estimated from the sum of Al, Si, Ca, Ti, and Fe after converting to their estimated oxide masses. "Smoke" was estimated from non-soil potassium by subtracting 0.6*Fe from the measured K values. The annual average values of these parameters were calculated from Götschi and colleagues [14] and are displayed in Fig. 15, in which the size of the pie chart is proportional to the annual average $PM_{2.5}$ mass concentration.

The highest mass concentrations are observed in northern Italy, where the chart for Verona has been omitted for clarity. In most locations, most of the composition was not measured. In southern Europe, a greater influence of "soil" is likely the result of frequent incursions of dust from the Sahara Desert. In northern Europe, there is more influence of transported ammonium sulfate.

Particle number concentrations

One of the major hypotheses proposed for the cause of the observed effect of PM on health is that high numbers of ultrafine particles (diameters

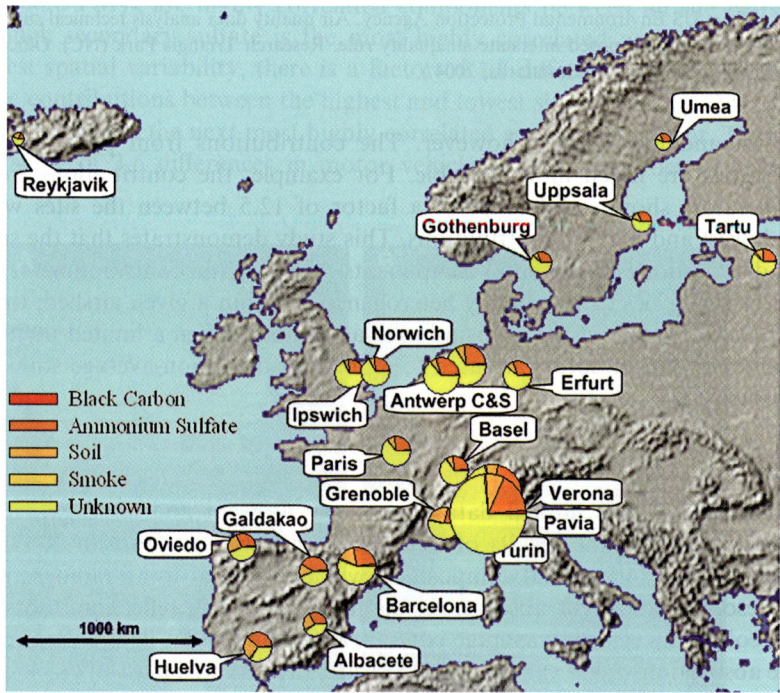

Fig. 15. Composition of $PM_{2.5}$ measured in 20 European cities by Götschi and colleagues [12] converted into composite variables using the approach of Malm and colleagues (1994). (*From* Götschi T, Hazenkamp-von Arx ME, Heinrich J, et al. Elemental composition and reflectance of ambient fine particles at 21 European locations. Atmos Environ 2005;39:5947–58; with permission.)

<0.1 μm) rather than particulate mass are important metric for exposure. Wichmann and colleagues [16] found significant associations of elevated cardiovascular and respiratory disease mortality with various fine (and ultrafine) particle indices evaluated in Erfurt, Germany. In this study, significant associations were found between mortality and ultrafine particle number concentration (NC), ultrafine particle mass concentration, fine particle mass concentration, and SO_2 concentration. The correlation between mass concentrations in the size range of 0.01 to 2.5 μm (mass concentration 0.01–2.5) and NC in the size range of 0.01 to 0.1 μm (NC0 0.01–0.1) was only moderate, which suggests that it may be possible to partially separate effects of ultrafine and fine particles. Measurements of the ultrafine particle concentrations and particle mass are needed to help provide more data to examine these relationships. There are few locations for which such data are available, however. In the Wichmann study, only particle counts were used. It is vital that we provide a clear record of the NC and size distributions of the ambient aerosol in the size range below a few hundreds of nanometers in particle diameter to provide critical data for evaluating the role of ultrafine particles in eliciting adverse health effects.

Because of the importance of particle effects on climate, there has been increased interest in the formation of particles in the ambient atmosphere. Evidence of nucleation has been observed in various places, including the free troposphere [17], the marine boundary layer [18], the vicinity of evaporating clouds [19], Arctic areas [20,21], urban areas and stack plumes [22], and boreal forests [23]. Similar events have been observed in Helsinki [24]. These events can be observed in terms of large numbers of small particles (often <0.010 μm in diameter). Even at 10 nm, we are able to infer the presence of nucleation events and particle growth in an urban area in which such data are rare.

There have been particle size measurements in Atlanta [25,26] and Pittsburgh [27]. Woo and colleagues [25] present the result of 13 months of measurements at a site in an industrial/commercial area northwest of downtown Atlanta. They found that particle NC tended to be higher on weekdays than on weekends. Concentrations of particles in the 10- to 100-nm and 100- to 2000-nm diameter ranges were higher at night than during the day and tended to reach their highest values during morning rush hour. Concentrations of 4 to 10 nm particles were elevated during rush hour when temperatures were <10°C. Annual average concentrations of particles in the 3- to 10-nm diameter range peak between 11 AM and 2 PM because of the appearance of high concentrations at those times on a few days. The results suggest that these high concentrations resulted from nucleation events and identify three types of "ultrafine particle" events. On days during August and April, pronounced peaks in the 3- to 10-nm size range occurred. These events typically occurred around noon, when solar radiation was high. During winter months, significantly elevated concentrations were seen in the 10- to 35-nm diameter range during the early morning and late afternoon hours. Relatively high NCs in the 35- to 45-nm diameter range also were detected several times. Elevated concentrations of SO_2 were observed during all three types of events. Nitrogen Oxides (NOx) were typically depleted during the 3- to 10-nm events and was more likely to be elevated during the 10- to 35-nm and 350 to 45-nm events. The sources of these particles are not yet known.

In Pittsburgh, 12 months of aerosol size distributions from 3 to 560 nm were measured using scanning mobility particle sizers from July 2001 to June 2002. The average Pittsburgh NC (3–500 nm) is 22,000 cm^{-3}, with an average mode size of 40 nm. Strong diurnal patterns in NC are evident as a direct effect of the sources of particles (atmospheric nucleation, traffic, and other combustion sources). New particle formation from homogeneous nucleation was observed to be significant on 30% to 50% of study days and over a wide area (at least 100 km). Rural NCs are a factor of two to three lower (on average) than the urban values.

The longest running series of measurements of particle size distributions in the United States was conducted in Rochester, New York. An initial summary of these results was provided by Jeong and colleagues [28]. More than 70% of total NC was associated with particles in the size range 0.011 to 0.05 µm, and approximately 20% was associated with particles 0.05 to 0.1 µm. Fig. 16 presents the annual variations of monthly average concentrations of ultrafine particles in the size range 0.011 to 0.050 µm. The mean

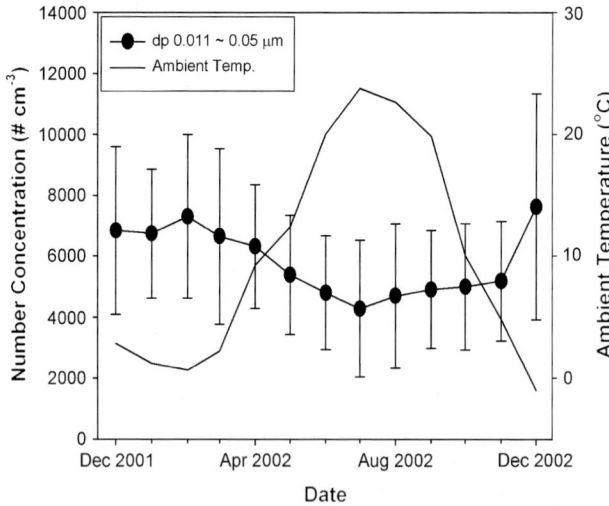

Fig. 16. Monthly variations of total NC and ambient temperature in Rochester, NY. (*From* Jeong CH, Hopke PK, Chalulpa D, et al. Characteristics of nucleation and growth events of ultrafine particles measured in Rochester, NY. Environ Sci Technol 2004;38:1933–40; with permission. © 2004 American Chemical Society.)

NC in the winter months, December to February, tended to be higher than the values in summer months, July to August. The highest mean NC (0.011–0.050 μm) was found during December 2002 with a mean of 7630 ± 3710 (mean ± standard deviation) cm^{-3}, whereas the lowest mean concentration was observed during July, with a value of 4280 ± 2250 cm^{-3}.

Two peaks in the NC were typically found in the size range of 0.011 to 0.05 μm as a function of time of day (Fig. 17). The first events occurred at approximately 8 AM During the winter months, these peaks were associated with increases in carbon monoxide. These particles seem to be from direct particle emissions from motor vehicles during the morning rush hour. Increases in this smallest size range particles also were observed in the late afternoon during the afternoon rush hour, particularly during the winter, when the mixing heights remain lower than during the summer. The second peak typically occurred between noon and 6 PM and was associated with nucleation events forming new ultrafine particles. These events were more likely in the spring and summer months. Sakurai and colleagues [29] have found that particles emitted by diesel engines include semivolatile and nonvolatile components. In the winter, the semivolatile material remains in the particulate phase, whereas in the summer there could be vaporization and loss of particle numbers.

Nucleation events are observed in the form of sharp increases in the concentrations of particles in the 0.011- to 0.050-μm size range. Peaks of SO$_2$ concentrations were observed during the nucleation events, whereas there

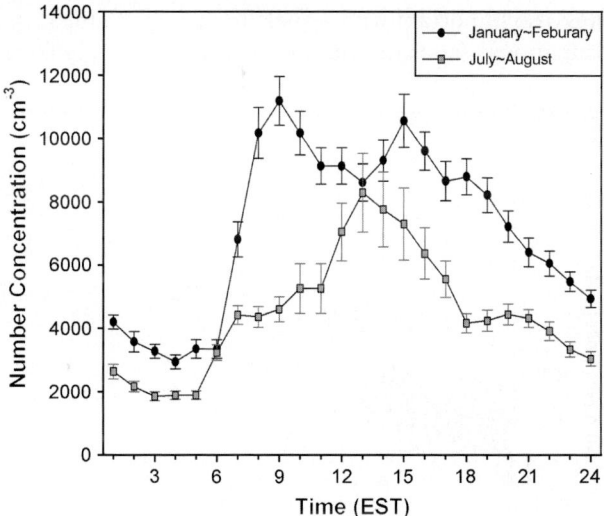

Fig. 17. Comparison of diurnal variations in ultrafine particles in the size range of 0.011 to 0.050 μm during winter months and summer months. (*From* Jeong CH, Hopke PK, Chalulpa D, et al. Characteristics of nucleation and growth events of ultrafine particles measured in Rochester, NY. Environ Sci Technol 2004;38:1933–40; with permission. © 2004 American Chemical Society.)

were no significant influences of $PM_{2.5}$ and carbon monoxide on the nucle-ation events. The increased SO_2 concentrations were observed when the wind direction was northwesterly, where large SO_2 sources were located. Re-searchers hypothesized that the ultrafine particles are sulfuric acid and water from the oxidation of SO_2. The relationship of NC in the 11- to 50-nm range and SO_2 is presented in Fig. 18. These events are assumed to be primarily associated with local SO_2 emissions.

There were also a more limited number of nucleation events followed by particle growth up to approximately 0.1 μm. These nucleation and growth events have been associated with regional events, as have been observed at several sites in Pennsylvania by Stanier and colleagues [27]. To have growth, there must be production of condensable vapor over a larger spatial domain. Researchers hypothesize that the larger domain provides adequate time to for photochemistry to convert volatile organic compounds into less volatile semi volatile organic compounds, which can then condense onto the particles and permit them to grow.

Exposure assessment of aerosols in occupational environments

Aerosol sampling in the workplace has evolved on a parallel course with ambient aerosol sampling, yet it is often more closely linked to the work process or task. As with ambient particles, size and shape are important in determining extent and location of deposition in the respiratory system and can be associated with disease. Another important distinction is that composition is also important with respect to damage to the respiratory sys-tem. The occupational exposure concentrations are often significantly higher

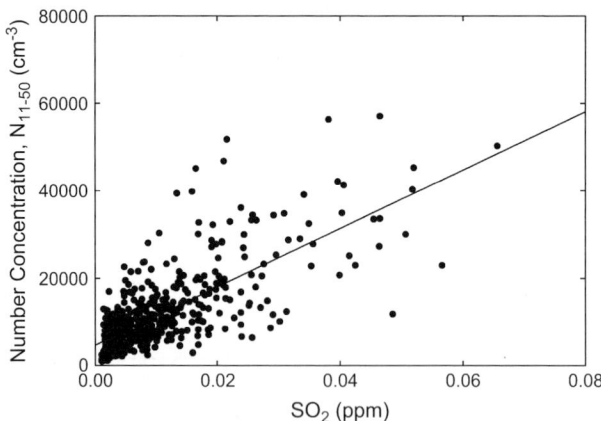

Fig. 18. Correlation between NC of ultrafine particles and SO_2 concentrations during the after-noon nucleation event from April to September 2002. (*From* Jeong CH, Hopke PK, Chalulpa D, et al. Characteristics of nucleation and growth events of ultrafine particles measured in Rochester, NY. Environ Sci Technol 2004;38:1933–40; with permission. © 2004 American Chemical Society.)

than in the ambient environment. Depending on the industrial process, the size may or may not be homogenous and the composition of the particulate may vary. The exposure assessment strategy must include the application of appropriate sampling and analytic techniques to ensure that worker exposure is adequately characterized by size, shape, and composition of the particulate. When comparing ambient aerosols to occupational aerosols, it is important to recognize that historically the particulate size terminology is somewhat different.

Occupational aerosols

Size selective sampling

A significant portion of the working population is exposed to elevated levels of aerosols. Dust, smoke, soot, mist fumes, and fogs are all types of aerosols generated in the work environment. Workplace exposure sampling can be traced back to the early 1900s, when mining and construction operations were evaluated for exposure to dusts that were associated with pneumoconiosis and other lung diseases [30]. These early sampling campaigns were focused on "total dust" ($d_{ae} < 100$ μm) and often overestimated exposure. As workplace sampling technology advanced, size selection for airborne PM became possible. The respirable ($d_{ae} < 10$ μm) or fine particulate fraction became possible to collect and was more closely linked with the risk of pneumoconiosis. As early as 1952, the British Medical Research Council defined "respirable dust" size fraction as PM capable of reaching the alveolar region of the lung. Organizations that formally established particle size-selective criteria early on were the US EPA [31] and the International Standards Organization [32], which determined three categories: inhalable, thoracic, and respirable fractions.

The American Conference of Governmental Industrial Hygienist has been establishing workplace exposure guidelines—referred to as threshold limit values—since 1946 and workplace particulate size-selective threshold limit values (TLVs) since the mid-1980s. The American Conference of Governmental Industrial Hygienist is a not-for-profit scientific association that proposes guidelines known as TLVs to be used in making decisions regarding acceptable levels of exposure to various airborne hazards found in the occupational environment. The particulate size-selective TLVs were established to address the association between illness and inhalation of particulate of certain size fractions. These workplace exposures are based on the assumption that for each substance there is some "safe or acceptable" level of exposure below which no significant adverse effects occur. The fractions of particulate established by the American Conference of Governmental Industrial Hygienist [33] are as follows:

1. Inhalable particulate mass TLVs are for materials that are hazardous when deposited anywhere in the respiratory tract and range in size from 0 to 100 μm in aerodynamic diameter.

2. Thoracic particulate mass TLVs are for materials that are hazardous when deposited in the lung airways and gas exchange region and range in size from 0 to 25 μm in aerodynamic diameter.
3. Respirable particulate mass TLVs are for materials that are hazardous when deposited in the gas exchange region and range in size from 0 to 10 μm in aerodynamic diameter.

The American Conference of Governmental Industrial Hygienist has recommended that airborne concentrations of respirable particles be kept below 3 mg/m^3 and below 10 mg/m^3 for inhalable particles unless a specific TLV has been established for the particular substance [33]. As an example, airborne samples of welding fume that contains metals such as lead, cadmium, nickel, or chromium would be compared with the specific TLV for the metal of concern and not to the size-selective particulate TLV.

Particulate composition

Although particulate size determines the deposition location in the respiratory system, composition of aerosols also can be important with respect to physiologic damage and subsequent disease. An effective exposure assessment may require air sampling for size-selective and process-specific type of aerosols [34]. A broad array of particulate contaminants is found in the work environment commonly ranging from 100 nm to 10 μm. Trace metals, crystalline silica, diesel particulate, metal working fluids, and asbestos fibers are several examples of occupational aerosols with specific toxic properties based on their composition. Although individual contaminants can exist, frequently a combination of aerosols results from a specific work environment. As an example, foundries, machining operations, and welding all result in aerosols containing particles of varying size with varying percentages of metals in the airborne sample. Individuals who work in an agricultural environment may be exposed to bioaerosols and disease particulate, which simultaneously may result in respiratory disease. These are just a few of the many types of aerosol exposures workers encounter on a routine basis; the effective characterization of workplace exposures often must include multiple sampling and analytic techniques to size select and analyze for various contaminants.

Exposure assessment in the workplace

Personal versus area sampling

Area sampling is helpful in determining sources of contamination and the general background exposure in a facility, yet generally it underestimates an individual exposure. When considering exposure assessment strategies for the work environment as opposed to the ambient air quality sampling, the most distinctive difference is the collection of personal samples versus area samples. The pattern of exposure of employees to hazardous agents is complicated by the mobility of employees and their interaction with the industrial process. Frequently there is large variability in concentration between locations within a facility, and the activities of employees cause additional variability because they often liberate contaminants into their breathing zone as they perform workplace tasks. The traditional characteristic of air contamination in an occupational environment is the continually changing concentration with respect to time and process. This factor means that air sampling must be performed in the breathing zone of the individual and spread over a sufficient time to characterize the individual's exposure adequately. This may be even more important with respect to aerosol sampling [35]. A personal breathing zone sample is collected within approximately 25 cm of the mouth and nose, which often is accomplished by attaching the sampler to the workers' lapels. This collection is done in an attempt to obtain a sample that closely approximates the concentration of contaminants a worker is breathing.

An implicit assumption associated with personal breathing zone samples is that the atmospheric concentration of the air contaminants at the lapel is equal to that inhaled by the worker. Although this is not always the case for aerosols, the size-selective sampling devices provide a means to better estimate exposure.

The fluctuations in airborne concentrations of contaminants during a work shift depend primarily on the process change over time, individual work practices, air turbulences, spills, and equipment failure. A personal sample on an individual allows one to capture the exposure of the individual during these dynamic events. It is usually not feasible to collect an air sample on every individual, however, and even if it were, daily assessments are not possible. Because of the inability to assess samples daily, an effective exposure assessment strategy must be established to characterize exposure to similarly exposed groups, such that effective controls can be prescribed for the entire workforce. In many cases, the risk to each individual can be estimated reliably by considering the exposure to a group of employees with similar working characteristics. Rarely do employees with the same job titles do the exact same activities; some care must be taken to assemble a group of workers into a similarly exposed group. The stratification of workers into similarly exposed groups allows for a more efficient allocation of resources and a characterization of exposures in the work environment [36].

Contemporary and emerging occupational aerosols

Key contemporary aerosol categories are summarized later to emphasize the broad span of industrial operations that generate aerosols and result in worker exposure. Although the list is large, a few key categories are reviewed later.

According to the National Science Foundation, the existing nanotechnology workforce numbers approximately 20,000, and the worldwide need will extend into several million workers in the next decade. Industry already has expressed a desire for trained workers at all levels, and states view nanotechnology as an area of investment that will make them economically viable. Nanoparticles are small enough to enter cells, which gives them the opportunity to interfere with the cells' biochemistry. They also can absorb ultraviolet light and trigger chemical reactions. Aerosol mass concentration is widely associated with health effects after inhalation; however, there is increasing evidence that mass concentration (mg/m^3) is a poor indicator of fine and ultrafine particle toxicity [37]. The risks associated with occupational exposures to nanoparticles have yet to be determined. Focused research is needed to understand the exposures and the corresponding health effects.

Trace metals, such as beryllium and cobalt, in aerodynamic diameters less than 2.5 are being evaluated with respect to dissolution of particles engulfed by macrophages. The mass-based occupational exposure limits have proved ineffective in reducing chronic beryllium disease [38]. The fine and ultrafine metal particulate may be a significant occupational health challenge as nanotechnology advances.

Background exposure to metal-working fluids has been associated with various respiratory diseases. Methods to measure liquid particulate, bioaerosol, and endotoxins associated with machining operations have been a continual challenge [39]. The liquid droplets present challenges with respect to size selection and quantification of exposure. The quantification of bioaerosol and, correspondingly, the meaning of the air sampling data with respect to health effects are other evolving areas.

Synthetic fibrous materials, such as refractory ceramic fibers that replaced asbestos in many applications, are an ongoing exposure interest. Associations between synthetic fibrous materials exposure and disease have been investigated by several researchers [40–43]. Fiber size and composition are of great interest with respect to exposure and disease, which requires continual evaluation to ensure that workers are adequately protected.

Particulate and gases

Indoor air pollutants are a complex matrix of continually interacting chemicals and particle species. Classes of contaminants such as PM_{10}, $PM_{2.5}$ and volatile organic compounds can have individual biologic impacts and interactions that can occur in the air and when they are inhaled. Current pollutant measurement systems only measure the predominant stable components of indoor air pollutants. Small amounts of more reactive chemicals not initially present in the air could result as the multiple compounds react and are inhaled. These reactive compounds could result in adverse health effects. Continued indoor air quality research is necessary to improve the exposure assessment capabilities in the indoor environment.

References

[1] US Environmental Protection Agency. Air quality criteria for particulate matter and sulfur oxides. Report no. EPA-600/8–82–029aF-cF. 3v. Research Triangle Park (NC): Office of Health and Environmental Assessment, Environmental Criteria and Assessment Office; 1982.

[2] US Environmental Protection Agency. Air quality criteria for particulate matter. Report no. EPA/600/P-95/001aF-cF. 3v. Research Triangle Park (NC): National Center for Environmental Assessment-RTP Office; 1996.

[3] US Environmental Protection Agency. Review of the national ambient air quality standards for particulate matter: policy assessment of scientific and technical information. Report no. EPA/452/R-96–013. Research Triangle Park (NC): Office of Air Quality Planning and Standards; 1996.

[4] European Union. Council directive 1999/30/EC of 22 April, 1999 relating to limit values for sulphur dioxide, nitrogen dioxide and oxides of nitrogen, particulate matter and lead in ambient air. Brussels: The Council of the European Union; 1999.

[5] US Environmental Protection Agency. Air quality data analysis technical support document for the proposed interstate air quality rule. Research Triangle Park (NC): Office of Air Quality Planning and Standards; 2004.

[6] Van Dingenen R, Raes F, Putaud JP, et al. A European aerosol phenomenology. I. Physical characteristics of particulate matter at kerbside, urban, rural and background sites in Europe. Atmos Environ 2004;36:2561–77.

[7] Health Effects Institute. Health effects of outdoor air pollution in developing countries of Asia: a literature review. Special Report 15. Boston (MA): Health Effects Institute; 2004.

[8] Smodis B. Applied environmental metrology for studying health-pollution interactions. J Radioanalytical and Nuclear Chemistry 2004;259:181–5.

[9] Hopke PK, Xie Y, Raunemaa T, et al. Characterization of Gent stacked filter unit PM10 sampler. Aerosol Sci Technol 1997;27:726–35.

[10] Begum BA, Biswas SK, Hopke PA. Temporal variations and spatial distribution of ambient PM2.2 and PM10 concentrations in Dhaka, Bangladesh. Sci Total Environ 2006;358(1-3): 36–45.

[11] Malm WC, Sisler JF, Huffman D, et al. Spatial and seasonal trends in particle concentration and optical extinction in the United States. J Geophys Res 1994;99:1347–70.

[12] Kim E, Hopke PK, Qin Y. Estimation of organic carbon blank values and error structures of the speciation trends network data for source apportionment. J Air Waste Manage Assoc 2005;55:1190–9.

[13] Kim E, Hopke PK, Pinto JP, et al. Spatial variability of fine particle mass, components, and source contributions during the regional air pollution study in St. Louis. Environ Sci Technol 2005;39:4172–9.

[14] Götschi T, Hazenkamp-von Arx ME, Heinrich J, et al. Elemental composition and reflectance of ambient fine particles at 21 European locations. Atmos Environ 2005;39: 5947–58.

[15] Cohen DD, Taha G, Stelcer E, et al. The measurement and sources of fine particle elemental carbon at several key sites in NSW over the past eight years. In: Proceedings of the 15th International Clean Air Conference. Mitcham, Victoria, Australia, November 27–30, 2000. pp. 485–490.

[16] Wichmann H-E, Spix C, Tuch T, et al. Daily mortality and fine and ultrafine particles in Erfurt, Germany. I. Role of particle number and particle mass. Cambridge (MA): Health Effects Institute; 2000.

[17] Raes F, Van Dingenen R, Cuevas E, et al. Observations of aerosols in the free troposphere and marine boundary layer of the subtropical Northeast Atlantic: discussion of process determining their size distributions. J Geophys Res 1997;102:21315–28.

[18] O'Dowd CD, Geever M, Hill MK, et al. New particle formation: nucleation rates and spatial scales in the clean marine coastal environment. Geophys Res Lett 1998;25:1661–4.

[19] Hegg DA, Radke LF, Hobbs PV. Measurements of Aitken nuclei and cloud condensation nuclei in the marine atmosphere and their relation to the DMS-cloud-climate hypothesis. J Geophys Res 1991;96:18727–33.

[20] Wiedensohler A, Covert DS, Swietlicki E, et al. Occurrence of an ultrafine particle mode less than 20 nm in diameter in the marine boundary layer during Arctic summer and autumn. Tellus 1996;48B:213–22.

[21] Pirjola L, Kulmala M. Modeling the formation of H_2SO_4 - H_2O particles in rural, urban, and marine conditions. Atmospheric Research 1998;46:321–47.

[22] Kerminen V, Wexler AS. The occurrence of sulfuric acid-water nucleation in plumes: urban environment. Tellus 1996;48B:65–82.

[23] Mäkelä JM, Aalto P, Jokinen V, et al. Observation of ultrafine aerosol particle formation and growth in boreal forest. Geophys Res Lett 1997;24:1219–22.

[24] Hussein T, Puustinen A, Aalto PP, et al. Urban aerosol number size distributions. Atmospheric Chemistry and Physics 2004;4:391–411.

[25] Woo KS, Chen DR, Pui DYH, et al. Measurement of Atlanta aerosol size distributions: observations of ultrafine particle events. Aerosol Sci Technol 2001;34:75–87.

[26] McMurry PH, Woo KS. Size distributions of 3–100 nm urban Atlanta aerosols: measurement and observations. J Aerosol Med 2002;15:169–78.

[27] Stanier C, Khlystov A, Pandis SN. Ambient aerosol size distributions and number concentrations measured during the Pittsburgh Air Quality Study (PAQS). Atmos Environ 2004;38: 3275–84.

[28] Jeong CH, Hopke PK, Chalulpa D, et al. Characteristics of nucleation and growth events of ultrafine particles measured in Rochester, NY. Environ Sci Technol 2004;38:1933–40.

[29] Sakurai H, Park K, McMurry PH, et al. Size-dependent mixing characteristics of volatile and nonvolatile components in diesel exhaust aerosols. Environ Sci Technol 2003;37: 5487–95.

[30] Walton WH, Vincent JH. Aerosol instrument in occupational hygiene: an historical perspective. Aerosol Science Technology 1998;28:417–38.

[31] Miller F, Gardner D, Graham J. Size considerations for establishing a standard for inhalable particles. J Air Pollut Control Assoc 1979;29:610–5.

[32] International Standards Organization. Air quality particle size fraction definitions for health-related sampling. Technical report ISO/TR/7708-1983(revised 1992). Geneva (Switzerland): International Standards Organization; 1983.

[33] American Conference of Governmental Industrial Hygienist. (2005) Threshold limit values for chemical substances and physical agents and biological exposure indices. Cincinnati (OH): American Conference of Governmental Industrial Hygienist; 2005. p. 74–5.

[34] Vincent JH. Sampling criteria for inhalable fraction. In: Vincent JH, editor. Particle size-selective sampling for particulate air contaminants. Cincinnati (OH): ACGIH Worldwide; 1999. p. 51–3.

[35] Rappaport S. Assessment of long-term exposure to toxic substances in air. Ann Occup Hyg 1991;35:61–121.

[36] Mulhausen JR, Damiano J. Strategy for assessing and managing occupational exposures. Fairfax (VA): AIHA; 1998. p. 1–39.

[37] Maynard A, Maynard R. A derived association between ambient aerosol surface area and excess mortality using historic time series data. Atmos Environ 2002;36:5561–7.

[38] Day G, Hoover M, Stefaniak A, et al. Bioavailability of beryllium oxide particles: an in vitro study in the murine j774a.1 macrophage cell line model. Exp Lung Res 2005;31(3): 341–60.

[39] Gorny R, Reponen T, Grinshpun S, et al. Source strength of fungal spore aerosolization from moldy building material. Atmos Environ 2004;35:4853–62.

[40] Lentz T, Rice C, Succop P, et al. Pulmonary deposition modeling with airborne fiber exposure data: a study of workers manufacturing refractory ceramic fibers. Appl Occup Environ Hyg 2003;18:278–88.

[41] Fayerweather W, Eastes W, Cereghini R, et al. Quantitative risk assessment of durable glass fibers. Inhal Toxicol 2002;14(6):553–68.

[42] Walker AM, Maxim LD, Utell M. Risk analysis for mortality from respiratory tumors in a cohort of refractory ceramic fiber workers. Regul Toxicol Pharmacol 2002;35(1):95–104.

[43] Lundgren DA, Burton RM. Effect of particle size distribution on the cut point between fine and coarse ambient mass fractions. In: Phalen RF, Bates DV, editors. Proceedings of the colloguium on particulate air pollution and human mortality and morbidity. Inhal Toxicol 1995;7:131–48.

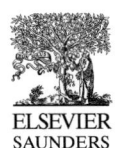

ELSEVIER
SAUNDERS

Clin Occup Environ Med
5 (4) 773–784

CLINICS IN
OCCUPATIONAL AND
ENVIRONMENTAL
MEDICINE

Aerosol Dosimetry Considerations

Robert F. Phalen, PhD[a,b,c,*],
Michael J. Oldham, PhD[a,b]

[a]Department of Community and Environmental Medicine, School of Medicine,
University of California, 100 FRF Building, Room 1,
North Campus, Irvine, CA 92697-1825, USA
[b]Air Pollution Health Effects Laboratory, University of California, Irvine,
CA 92697-1825, USA
[c]Center for Occupational and Environmental Health, University of California,
Irvine, CA 92697-1830, USA

Dose considerations are among the most fundamental concepts of toxicology, and inhalation toxicology is no exception; expression of the full-range of possible effects—from no effects (or beneficial effects) to adverse effects to fatal effects—is seen to unfold as the dose is increased for essentially all inhaled substances. Dose-response considerations are key in establishing permissible exposures in occupational and nonoccupational environments.

Even when the exposures are identical, some individuals (or groups of individuals) receive larger or smaller doses than those received by the average person. It is reasonable to expect that individuals/groups that receive the greatest doses are also at greater risk. High-dose and high-risk groups are sometimes referred to as "potentially sensitive subpopulations." It is clear that dose alone does not explain all adverse responses, because concurrent illness, genetic makeup, exposure history, and other factors modify susceptibility.

Defining "dose" for inhaled aerosol particles

For inhaled particles, the concept of dose can be relatively complicated in that it may relate to several quantities. The exposure dose (D_e) is

$$D_e = C \bullet T \tag{1}$$

This article was supported by the Charles C. Stocking Family Trust via an endowment.

* Corresponding author. Department of Community and Environmental Medicine, School of Medicine, University of California, 100 FRF Building, Room 1, North Campus, Irvine, CA 92697-1825.

E-mail address: rfphalen@uci.edu (R.F. Phalen).

doi:10.1016/j.coem.2006.07.004
occmed.theclinics.com

in which C is the average airborne aerosol concentration (eg, particle mass or count per unit volume of air or other relevant metric) and T is the duration of exposure. The inhaled dose (D_i) is

$$D_i = C \bullet T \bullet V_m \bullet I \tag{2}$$

in which V_m is the ventilation per unit time and I is the inhalability (sampling efficiency of the nose/mouth). The total deposited dose (D_d) is

$$D_d = C \bullet T \bullet V_m \bullet I \bullet DF_t \tag{3}$$

in which DF_t is the total respiratory tract deposition fraction. The regional deposited dose (D_r) is

$$D_r = C \bullet T \bullet V_m \bullet I \bullet DF_r \tag{4}$$

in which DF_r is the deposition fraction in the region of interest (eg, nose, tracheobronchial tree, or pulmonary zone). The amount deposited per unit surface area in the region of interest D_{rsa} is

$$D_{rsa} = C \bullet T \bullet V_m \bullet I \bullet DF_r/S_r \tag{5}$$

in which S_r is the surface area of the region of interest.

For the purposes of understanding the health effects of inhaled particles, equations (4) and (5) are usually the most important. Simpler concepts of dose, such as that described in equation (1), are often used in toxicology and epidemiology, however. When the inhalability, deposition fractions, and surface areas are included in dosimetry considerations, the aid of a specialist trained in inhalation toxicology is useful.

In this article, fundamental concepts of aerosol dosimetry and some applications related to the health effects of inhaled particles are considered. The topics covered include useful definitions, including the aerodynamic diameter of aerosol particles, how inhaled particles deposit in the human respiratory tract, models for calculating inhaled aerosol deposition, factors that increase aerosol deposition doses (eg, exercise, body size, and respiratory disease), and particle clearance. Some current challenges, unsolved problems, and speculations related to inhaled aerosol dosimetry also are presented.

Aerosol basics

Useful definitions

An aerosol is a two-phase system that consists of finely divided condensed matter (solids or liquids) suspended in a gas, which is usually air

(which also includes co-pollutant gases and vapors). The essential characteristic of an aerosol system is that it is relatively time-stable. That is, the suspended particles do not rapidly settle out of the suspending gas. This
characteristic limits the upper size of particles that can exist in an aerosol.
Particles with diameters (aerodynamic diameters) that are larger than
100 μm settle out rapidly and are the largest particles that are generally considered by aerosol scientists. The lower limit of particle size is less clearly
defined. When particles are smaller than approximately 0.001 μm in
diameter (geometric diameter), they contain so few atoms and have such
large surface-to-volume ratios that they tend to evaporate and re-form in
the air. The particle diameter range of 0.001 to 100 μm is usually considered
by aerosol scientists. This broad size range covers four regimes in physics:
the free-molecule regime (in which diffusion dominates particle motion),
the continuum regime (in which gravitational forces and particle inertia
dominate motion), and two intermediate regimes (which are transitional
with respect to particle motion).

The aerodynamic diameter (D_{ae}) is an important concept in inhalation
toxicology. The aerodynamic diameter (also the aerodynamic equivalent diameter) is the physical diameter of a smooth sphere with a density of 1 g/cm^3
that has the same terminal settling velocity in still air (under standard laboratory conditions) as the particle in question. For example, a solid gold
smooth spherical particle with a physical diameter of 1 μm has an aerodynamic diameter of approximately 4.4 μm because of the density of gold
(19.3 g/cm^3). For smooth spheres $D_{ae} = D_p \bullet (P_p)^{1/2}$, in which D_p is the
physical diameter, and ρ_p is the particle density. The aerodynamic diameter
of a particle influences several important kinetic properties, such as its settling rate and inertial behavior when in motion.

Particle motion

To understand the deposition efficiencies of inhaled aerosol particles,
a consideration of particle motion is helpful. Table 1 shows the rate of
movement of particles in still air and the time required to travel 1 cm
(T_{1cm}) from an original release point.

Consider a person inhaling the various particles in Table 1 in which movement away from the inhaled air stream by even a fraction of a centimeter may
cause the particles to touch an airway wall and deposit (the sticking coefficient
for a particle touching an airway surface = 1; that is, if it touches, it sticks). It is
clear that the smallest particles depart the air stream and deposit by diffusion,
and the largest particles deposit by sedimentation (and by inertial motion,
which is related to particle mass). The net result is that inhaled particle deposition efficiency curves are U-shaped (ie, the large and the small particles have
high deposition efficiencies, and particles between 0.1 and 1.0 μm in diameter
have the lowest deposition efficiencies). A minimum in the total respiratory
tract deposition efficiency occurs for particles that are approximately 0.3 μm

Table 1
Movement of spherical particles of density 1 g/cm^3 and the time required for a displacement of 1 cm in still air

Diameter (μm)	Settling velocity (cm/s)	Diffusion velocity (cm/s)	T_{1cm} via settling	T_{1cm} via diffusion
100	25	6.9×10^{-5}	0.04 sec	4 h
10	0.31	2.2×10^{-4}	3.2 sec	76 min
1	3.5×10^{-3}	7.4×10^{-3}	4.7 min	23 min
0.1	8.6×10^{-5}	3.7×10^{-3}	3.2 h	4.5 min
0.01	6.7×10^{-6}	3.3×10^{-2}	1.7 d	30 sec
0.001	6.5×10^{-7}	0.32	18 d	3.1 sec

Data from Hinds WC. Aerosol technology. 2nd edition. New York: John Wiley and Sons; 1999. p. 459.

in diameter; under ordinary resting conditions more than 80% of these inhaled particles typically are exhaled without depositing.

Inhaled particle deposition and clearance

Inhaled particle deposition curves

Inhaled particle deposition curves describe the probability of deposition of inhaled particles as a function of particle diameter. One such curve, for an adult man performing light work (10 L/min ventilation), is shown in Fig. 1A [1]. Four curves are shown, one for total deposition (anywhere in the respiratory tract), one for deposition in the nose/oral cavity/pharynges/larynx, one for deposition in the tracheobronchial region, and one for deposition in the alveolarized, pulmonary (P) region. Although the four curves are not simple, each has a minimum deposition efficiency somewhere between 0.1 and 1.0 μm diameter particles. Each of the four curves also has a peak on either side of the minimum, which is produced by the effects of diffusion, sedimentation, and impaction. Equation (2) introduced the concept of inhalability, which relates to the fact that large particles are difficult to inhale (because they are settling out of the air entering the nose or mouth). Fig. 1B shows inhaled deposition curves as corrected for inhalability [1]. Note that 100 μm diameter particles are only 50% inhalable, as seen by their total deposition efficiency changing from 100% in Fig. 1A to 50% in Fig. 1B. These curves, which have been obtained by many clinical measurements and mathematical modeling [2,3], apply only to the standard man.

Many factors have an effect on the inhaled particle deposition curves; level of exercise, age, body size, respiratory disease, and even normal population variability (in anatomy or physiology) shift the curves one way or another. Fortunately, it is not necessary to have hundreds of such curves on hand, because computer software is available to perform inhaled particle deposition calculations for nearly all cases of interest [2,4,5]. The software MPPD1 is particularly useful, because it is free (from CIIT, 2005), covers

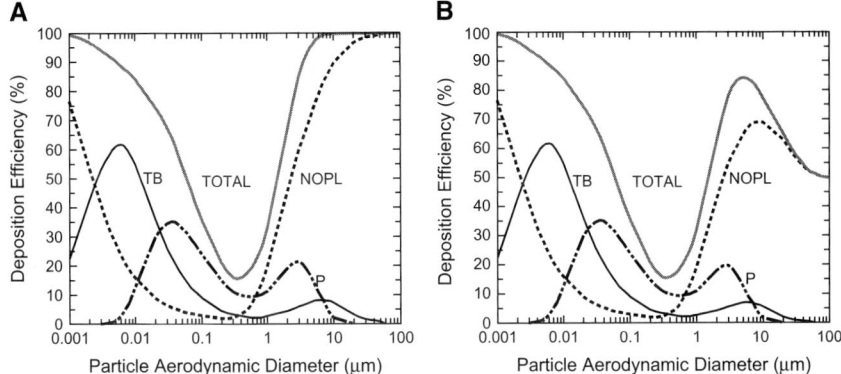

Fig. 1. Particle deposition curves in the average adult man. NOPL, naso-oro-pharyngo-laryngeal region; TB, tracheobronchial region; P, pulmonary region. Part A is uncorrected for inhalability, and part B is corrected for inhalability. (*From* Phalen RF. The particulate air pollution controversy. Boston: Kluwer Academic Publishers; 2002. p. 60; with kind permission of Springer Science and Business Media.)

humans and rats, allows input of particle size distribution data, age, ventilation, and other important variables, and is relatively user-friendly.

Local particle deposition hot spots

The preceding information relates to averaged deposition doses in the respiratory tract or specific regions, such as the nasal, tracheobronchial, or alveolarized airways. For many purposes, such averaged doses are sufficient. If local doses (eg, within portions of bronchial tubes) are of interest, however, different models and more detailed laboratory measurements must be consulted. There is a great deal of convincing evidence that inhaled particle deposition is nonuniform. The analysis of mammalian lung samples shows that particles deposit and are retained preferentially at thousands of points in the respiratory tract, especially at the bifurcating regions of the tracheobronchial airways [6–8]. The locations and intensities of these hot spots of particle deposition have been modeled successfully using computational fluid dynamics techniques [9–13]. Depending on the size of the hot spot, local dose enhancement factors of 100 or more over the doses to nearby surfaces are seen. Although the health significance of these high local doses is still uncertain, it is likely that in some individuals their impact on adverse health outcomes may be significant. Such hot spots also have implications for particle doses used in in vitro toxicology studies.

Other factors that may increase inhaled particle doses

Healthy and diseased individuals can belong to subpopulations that receive greater than average doses from inhaled particles. These high-dose

subpopulations include (1) otherwise normal people who have airway anat-
omies/breathing characteristics that are extreme in the healthy population
distribution, (2) very young, very small, or obese individuals (who have
high V_m in relation to their lung sizes), (3) people who have lung diseases
that produce uneven airflow patterns, (4) people who are engaged in exercise, (5) people with impaired particle clearance, and (6) people who are exposed in close proximity to local particle sources. The inhaled particle
deposition curves shown in Fig. 1 actually represent population averages,
and some members of the population have much greater deposition efficiencies than the average individual [14]. In these individuals, factors of two or
even three multiples of the average particle deposition may be seen. These
high-dose individuals are expected to potentially be at higher risk than are
individuals with average or lower doses.

The effects of age and body size on inhaled particle deposition can be significant. It is well known that smaller mammals tend to have higher ventilation rates per unit body mass (because of increased metabolism as a result of
loss of body heat) than normal sized individuals. Newborns and neonates,
for example, can have inhaled particle deposition rates in the tracheobronchial region per kilogram of body mass that are nearly ten times greater than
that for adults [15,16], and obesity can lead to even greater particle deposition in children [17].

Exercise can increase greatly the volume of air inhaled per unit time and
nearly proportionately increase particle doses. Various states of exertion can
increase the rate of intake of air by large amounts, as shown in Table 2.

Lung diseases, such as chronic obstructive pulmonary disease and
asthma, can increase the deposition doses from inhaled particles in several

Table 2
Body mass, height, and minute ventilation at three levels of activity for selected ages

| Age (y) | Mass (kg) | Height (cm) | Minute Ventilation (L)[a] | | |
			Low activity	Light exercise	Heavy exercise
0	3.3	50	1.5	3.0	8.9
2	13.0	88	2.8	5.5	16.4
4	16.4	104	3.2	6.3	19.0
6	22.0	115	3.9	7.8	23.2
8	27.0	127	4.5	9.1	27.1
10	34.0	138	5.4	10.8	32.4
12	43.0	150	6.6	13.1	39.3
14	54.0	162	8.0	15.9	47.8
16	63.0	170	9.1	18.2	54.6
18	70.0	175	10.0	20.0	60.0

[a] Terminology used for describing ventilation is arbitrary because no standard accepted
definitions exist.

Adapted from Phalen RF, Oldham MJ, Kleinman MT, et al. Tracheobronchial deposition
predictions for infants, children and adolescents. Ann Occup Hyg 1988;32(Suppl 1):11–21;
with permission of the Oxford University Press.

ways; they can increase the total volume of air inhaled for a given level of physical activity, they can decrease the portion of the lung that is ventilated, and they can greatly increase the nonuniformity of particle deposition [18–22]. These factors combine to place persons with lung disease in the unfavorable category of a high-dose plus a potentially high-risk subpopulation.

Impaired particle clearance, in general, does not increase the initial deposition doses, but it does increase the integrated doses to those tissues that have slow particle clearance rates. The three main factors associated with impaired clearance are (1) normal variations in clearance rates, (2) acute infections, such as influenza, and (3) chronic diseases that are associated with poor particle clearance [23–25]. Persons with poor particle clearance usually augment normal clearance mechanisms with coughing. Coughing fits, which are characterized by numerous rapid coughs separated by long intervals of eupnea, can effectively move mucus and trapped particles up the airways generation by generation to a point at which they are swallowed. As a rule of thumb, each cough can be expected to move mucus accumulations upward one generation, which is why coughing fits are required to eliminate deeply lying mucus.

Another important factor that increases particle deposition relates to exposure in close proximity to particle sources. For example, exposure downwind from and near busy roads—or other areas of high particle concentrations—can lead to exposures that are significantly greater than would be expected on the basis of central air monitoring data [26,27]. Likewise, exposures that take place near certain industrial sources, construction sites, or during some personal activities (eg, vacuuming, composting, smoking, wood working) can significantly increase personal exposures.

Controlling doses in high-risk individuals

If one considers the simultaneous occurrence of several of the foregoing exposure factors, it is easy to envision the highest risk individuals. For example, a young or overweight person with chronic obstructive lung disease (or another lung disease) who also has an acute respiratory tract infection, is engaged in exercise, and is exposed near a busy road can receive enormous doses in comparison to the average individual. Attempting to protect such rare, but unlucky, individuals by tightening regional air standards may be difficult, unduly expensive (in terms of direct costs and indirect economic impacts), or simply impossible. For this reason, high air pollution alerts that encourage individual protective behavioral changes probably always will be needed. Such behavioral changes include curtailing physical activity, seeking cleaner environments (eg, air-conditioned structures), reducing certain personal activities that generate pollutants, using indoor air cleaners, and even taking doctor-recommended medications that prevent significant or life-threatening responses (eg, acute asthma attacks).

Challenges and unsolved problems

Although much is known regarding the dosimetry of inhaled particles, various significant challenges remain. Most importantly, it is still difficult to predict individual exposures confidently. Most of the scientific knowledge and available particle dosimetry software relates to normal individuals. Certainly, a high priority for research is to increase the database to include the effects of age, body size, and disease states on inhaled particle doses and to incorporate this information into the available dosimetry software. Similarly, more information on personal exposures, as opposed to reliance on fixed aerosol monitors, is needed. Progress in this area requires the development of inexpensive, lightweight particle monitors that can be comfortably worn for long periods by potentially high-risk subpopulations and individuals. More data are needed to better define the full range of personal activities that generate excessive particle exposures.

A serious complication in defining particle exposures relates to defining the proper dose metrics. A useful dose metric is one that measures the important (ie, mechanistically associated with adverse health effects) properties of inhaled particles in a reliable reproducible manner. Several particle properties have been considered with respect to the dose metrics. Particle mass within a defined particle size range is most commonly used, but particle count, particle surface area, and particle chemistry are also recognized as being important in certain circumstances [1]. Probably any measurable particle property (eg, size, mass, count, surface area, aspect ratio, fractal dimension, acidity, oxidative capacity, solubility, and catalytic activity) has some potentially adverse impact on some people. The presence of gaseous/vaporous co-pollutants cannot be ignored. Considerable sustained research is needed to define and evaluate the many potential dose metrics. Only when such research is substantially completed will it be possible to confidently propose effective and cost-efficient air quality regulations.

Challenges also exist with respect to defining and using better laboratory animal models for aerosol toxicity research. Several advances in developing health-compromised animal models have been valuable [28–35], but establishing their relationships to human diseases remains problematic. An important issue with all laboratory animals relates to species differences in particle deposition and clearance [1]. Great care must be taken in selecting such models, but they are clearly essential for conducting particle toxicity studies.

To improve the quality of data that are available for epidemiologic analyses, information on body mass and height, physical activity patterns, lifestyle factors (eg, smoking status), health status, place of residence (eg, urban or rural), personal activities and hobbies, and other dosimetry-related data should be collected, as should the usual demographic descriptors (eg, gender, age, education, and income). The quality of epidemiologic findings is enhanced by defining more clearly the (often rare) individuals in potentially susceptible subpopulations who are at significant risk of experiencing the adverse effects of exposures to particles. From a clearer understanding of dose-response associations among high-risk individuals, it will be more feasible to devise appropriate public health interventions for protection of high-risk subpopulations from the effects of exposures to particles.

A particularly interesting problem related to dose-response relationships is that for a given dose, the response can depend on the previous recent exposure history. Previous exposure, or lack thereof, alternatively can produce either adaptation or sensitization. For example, in short-term time series epidemiologic studies, statistically significant responses are often associated with increases, or increments, in particle concentrations, as opposed to levels of particles [36]. For example, associations (between adverse outcomes and particle measures) are seen when 3- to 5-day averages in particle concentrations are used as measures of exposure. This implies that previous exposure to cleaner air may intensify the adverse effects on some (perhaps many) individuals. Why this might occur is unclear; perhaps short-term loss of normal defenses is occurring. Although this issue is not strictly a dosimetry problem, it relates to how dose is interpreted. Possible long-term adaptation to aerosols and the potential physiologic costs of such require additional research.

An unsettled area in inhalation toxicology and dosimetry research involves the health effects of low doses (minimally polluted air). Specifically, can the effects of such low doses be extrapolated from observations at moderate doses? Can the air actually be too clean, in that exposed populations may be unable to tolerate future unavoidable higher particle exposures? Are low levels of air pollutants even beneficial to overall health, as related to possible hormetic effects [37]? A recently introduced scientific journal, *Dose-Respones* [38], publishes papers related to low-dose exposures and their effects.

Summary

Dosimetric considerations are clearly essential to an adequate understanding of the health effects of inhaled particulate air pollutants. Defining exposure in terms of C • T is not adequate, because it ignores such important factors as volume of air inspired, aerosol inhalability, deposition efficiency, uniformity of deposition, local deposition intensities (eg, deposited dose per unit surface area), and the actions of particle clearance/redistribution mechanisms. By considering these and other potentially important dose-related factors, it may be possible to identify high-risk individuals within potentially susceptible subpopulations. When an individual is at high risk (because of disease or genetic or exposure history factors) and receives unusually high doses (because of anatomic, physiologic, and environmental factors), he or she is likely to be the most severely harmed. Some of the factors that predispose individuals to receiving high doses and being at high risk are identified, and others are still under investigation. It is important that these factors be more thoroughly incorporated into epidemiologic and human clinical investigations, so that individuals most severely affected can be identified clearly and protected appropriately. Otherwise, increasingly restrictive and costly particle control strategies may be pursued without significant net benefits to public health.

Research intended to identify the more harmful particulate agents, combinations, and temporal exposure effects requires the use of laboratory animal models in the foreseeable future. Understanding species differences in particle deposition and clearance is fundamental to the use of such investigations. More is known about species differences in healthy animals than in health-compromised ones. Additional research on such compromised animal models is needed.

Difficult problems remain in understanding the effects of low doses and the effects of mixtures and intermittent high- and low-level exposures. Until more is learned about these problems, it is difficult to have confidence in the effects of control strategies based on finding acceptable air concentrations of air pollutants one by one.

Current coordinated research efforts are underway worldwide to better understand the potential adverse health effects of current particle exposures. The Committee on Research Priorities for Airborne Particulate Matter of the National Research Council has defined many important issues (including dosimetric ones) and a logical sequence of research activities to better understand them [39]. The identified National Research Council research agenda is a long-term proposition that provides important guidance to many research communities.

Acknowledgments

Susan Akhavan provided manuscript production and editing, and James Enstrom and Robert Friis contributed critical comments.

References

[1] Phalen RF. The particulate air pollution controversy. Boston: Kluwer Academic Publishers; 2002. p. 55–64, 69–80.

[2] International Commission on Radiological Protection. Human respiratory tract model for radiological protection (ICRP publication 66). Tarrytown (NY): Elsevier Science; 1994.

[3] National Council on Radiation Protection and Measurements. Deposition, retention and dosimetry of inhaled radioactive substances (NCRP report 125). Bethesda (MD): National Council on Radiation Protection and Measurements; 1997.

[4] CIIT. CIIT Centers for Health Technology Transfer. Available at: www.ciit.org/mppd/. Accessed August 28, 2005.

[5] Brown JS, Wilson WF, Grant LD. Dosimetric comparisons of particle deposition and retention in rats and humans. Inhal Toxicol 2005;17(7–8):355–85.

[6] Ishikawa Y, Nakagawa K, Satoh Y, et al. Hot spots of chromium accumulation at bifurcations of chromate workers' bronchi. Cancer Res 1994;54(9):2342–6.

[7] Kaye SB, Phillips CG, Winlove CP. Measurement of non-uniform aerosol deposition patterns in the conducting airways of the porcine lung. J Aerosol Sci 2000;31(7):849–66.

[8] Schlesinger RB, Gurman JL, Lippmann M. Particle deposition within bronchial airways: comparisons using constant and cyclic inspiratory flows. Ann Occup Hyg 1982;26(1–4): 47–64.

[9] Gradón L, Orlinki D. Deposition of inhaled aerosol particles in a generation of the tracheobronchial tree. J Aerosol Sci 1990;21(1):3–19.

[10] Balásházy I, Farkas A, Hofmann W, et al. Local deposition distributions of inhaled radionuclides in the human tracheobronchial tree. Radiat Protect Dosimetry 2002;99(1–4): 469–70.

[11] Hofmann W, Balásházy I, Heistracher T, et al. The significance of particle deposition patterns in bronchial airway bifurcations for extrapolation modeling. Aerosol Sci Technol 1996;25(3):305–27.

[12] Zhang Z, Kleinstreuer C, Donohue JF, et al. Comparison of micro- and nano-size particle depositions in a human upper airway model. J Aerosol Sci 2005;36(2):211–33.

[13] Oldham MJ, Phalen RF, Heistracher T. Computational fluid dynamic predictions and experimental results for particle deposition in an airway model. Aerosol Sci Technol 2000; 32(1):61–71.

[14] Lippmann M. Regional deposition of particles in the human respiratory tract. In: Lee DHK, Falk HL, S.D., et al, editors. Handbook of physiology: reactions to environmental agents. Bethesda (MD): American Physiological Society; 1977. p. 213–32.

[15] Phalen RF, Oldham MJ, Kleinman MT, et al. Tracheobronchial deposition predictions for infants, children and adolescents. Ann Occup Hyg 1988;32(Suppl 1):11–21.

[16] Phalen RF, Oldham MJ, Dunn-Rankin D. Inhaled particle mass per unit body mass per unit time. Appl Occup Environ Hyg 1992;7(4):246–52.

[17] Bennett WD, Zeman KL. Effect of body size on breathing pattern and fine particle deposition in children. J Appl Physiol 2004;97(3):821–6.

[18] Chalupa DC, Morrow PE, Oberdorster G, et al. Ultrafine particle deposition in subjects with asthma. Environ Health Perspect 2004;112(8):879–82.

[19] Bennett WD. How may the dosimetry of inhaled particles play a role in the observed mortality/morbidity associated with PM10. Inhal Toxicol 2000;12(Suppl 1):33–6.

[20] Brown JS, Zeman KL, Bennett WD. Regional deposition of coarse particles and ventilation distribution in healthy subjects and patients with cystic fibrosis. J Aerosol Med 2001;14(4): 443–54.

[21] Kim CS, Khang TC. Comparative measurement of lung deposition of inhaled fine particles in normal subjects and patients with obstructive airway disease. Am J Respir Crit Care Med 1997;155(3):899–905.

[22] Sweeney TD, Skornik WA, Brain JD, et al. Chronic-bronchitis alters the pattern of aerosol deposition in the lung. Am J Crit Care Med 1995;151(2):482–8.

[23] Pavia D, Bateman JRM, Clarke SW. Deposition and clearance of inhaled particles. Bull Eur Physiopath Resp 1980;16(3):355–66.

[24] Pavia D. Acute respiratory infections and mucociliary clearance. Eur J Respir Dis 1987; 71(4):219–26.

[25] Smaldone GC, Foster WM, Oriordan TG, et al. Regional impairment of mucociliary clearance in chronic obstructive pulmonary disease. Chest 1993;103(5):1390–6.

[26] Zhu Y, Hinds WC, Kim S, et al. Concentration and size-distribution of ultrafine particles near a major highway. J Air Waste Manage Assoc 2002;52(9):1032–42.

[27] Chang LT, Koutrakis P, Catalano PJ, et al. Hourly personal exposures to fine particles and gaseous pollutants: results from Baltimore, Maryland. J Air Waste Manage Assoc 2000; 50(7):1223–35.

[28] Bice DE, Seagrave JC, Green FHY. Animal models of asthma: potential usefulness for studying health effects of inhaled particles. Inhal Toxicol 2000;12(9):829–62.

[29] Cantor JO, editor. CRC handbook of animal models of pulmonary disease. Boca Raton (FL): CRC Press; 1989.

[30] Conn CA, Green FHY, Nikula KJ. Animal models of pulmonary infection in the compromised host: potential usefulness for studying health effects of inhaled particles. Inhal Toxicol 2000;12(9):783–827.

[31] Mauderly JL. Animal models for the effect of age on susceptibility to inhaled particulate matter. Inhal Toxicol 2000;12(9):863–900.

[32] Muggenburg BA, Tilley L, Green FHY. Animal models of cardiac disease: potential usefulness for studying health effects of inhaled particles. Inhal Toxicol 2000;12(9):901–25.

[33] Utell MJ, Frampton MW. Who is susceptible to particulate matter and why? Inhal Toxicol 2000;12(Suppl 1):37–40.

[34] Miller FJ, Anjilvel S, Ménache MG, et al. Dosimetric issues relating to particulate toxicology. Inhal Toxicol 1995;7(5):615–32.

[35] Costa DL, Kodavanti UP. Toxic responses of the lung to inhaled pollutants: benefits and limitations of lung disease models. Toxicol Lett 2003;140(Special issue):195–203.

[36] Pope CA III. Epidemiology of fine particulate air pollution and human health: biologic mechanisms and who's at risk? Environ Health Perspect 2000;108(10):A713–23.

[37] Calabrese EJ. Hormetic dose-responses relationships in immunology: occurrence, quantitative features of the dose-response, mechanistic foundations, and clinical implications. Crit Rev Toxicol 2005;35(2–3):35–89.

[38] Dose-Response. Available at: www.dose-response.com. Accessed August 28, 2006.

[39] NRC Committee on Research Priorities for Airborne Particulate Matter. Research priorities for airborne particulate matter: continuing research progress. Washington, DC: National Academies Press; 2004.

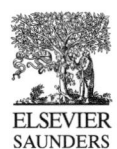

ELSEVIER
SAUNDERS

Clin Occup Environ Med
5 (4) 785–796

CLINICS IN
OCCUPATIONAL AND
ENVIRONMENTAL
MEDICINE

Translocation and Effects of Ultrafine Particles Outside of the Lung

Alison Elder, PhD*, Günter Oberdörster, DVM, PhD

Department of Environmental Medicine, University of Rochester,
575 Elmwood Avenue, Box 850, Rochester, NY 14642, USA

Epidemiologic studies have linked exposure to ambient particulate matter (PM) with respiratory and cardiovascular morbidity and mortality in susceptible parts of the population [1–7]. Controlled clinical studies with particles below 100 nm in diameter, termed ultrafine particles (UFP) or nanoparticles, have shown effects of exposure on blood leukocyte adhesion molecule expression, cardiac repolarization, and heart rate variability [8,9]. Studies in various animal susceptibility models exposed to laboratory surrogate UFP and freshly generated or concentrated ambient particles have shown mild but significant inflammatory responses in the lung [10–14] and extrapulmonary effects resulting in changes in blood coagulability, atherosclerotic plaque formation, leukocyte activation and surface adhesion molecule expression, heart tissue antioxidant gene expression, and heart rate variability [12,15–20].

Questions remain, however, regarding causal links between exposure and outcome and the mechanisms that control response. Ambient PM is comprised of four size fractions [21]. Ultrafine and smaller particles are formed in the vapor phase from a combination of anthropogenic and natural sources via nucleation and condensation processes. An important determinant of response for inhaled PM is the site of deposition. According to an International Commission on Radiological Protection predictive model [22], UFP deposit via diffusion with high efficiency in the alveolar regions of the lung, peaking at approximately 20 nm; particles between 5 and 20 nm deposit in all regions of the lung, including the nose. The fate of particles after

---

This article is adapted from Oberdörster G. Kinetics of inhaled ultrafine particles in the organism. In: Heinrich U (editor). Effects of air contaminants on the respiratory tract: interpretations from molecular to meta analysis. Stuttgart: Fraunhofer IRB Verlag; 2004. p. 121.

* Corresponding author.
E-mail address: alison_elder@urmc.rochester.edu (A. Elder).

doi:10.1016/j.coem.2006.07.003
occmed.theclinics.com

deposition is also important and translocation of deposited PM out of the lung represents one way in which clearance occurs. UFP, and presumably nanoparticles, are inefficiently cleared by resident macrophages from sites of deposition in the alveoli [23] and are retained on the epithelial surface to a greater degree than are larger particles. In turn, this greater retention potentially increases the possibility that ultrafine and smaller particles will be endocytosed by epithelial cells and translocated beyond their deposition site. Expanding on a previously published review, we explore the process of translocation as one mechanistic explanation for the observed adverse effects in susceptible individuals [24].

Deposition of ultrafine particles in the respiratory tract and translocation to extrapulmonary sites

Aside from deposition site, a critical determinant of response is the deposited dose. The dosimetry of inhaled PM is reviewed in the article by Phalen and Oldham in this issue. There are, however, nuances regarding UFP dosimetry that bear emphasis. An example in Fig. 1 shows the regional deposition of inhaled polydisperse 20-nm particles. The predicted deposited dose [25] in the three main regions of the respiratory tract is shown in terms of region and surface area. Although there are "hot spots" elsewhere, the UFP mass deposition is at a maximum in the alveolar regions of the lung. The epithelial surface area of the alveolar region is large compared with the upper airways, however; therefore, the UFP dose deposited per unit surface area is at a minimum in the alveoli. Despite the fact that UFP mass concentration in ambient air is low, UFP have the highest number concentration of the size fractions and can be up to 60,000 times more

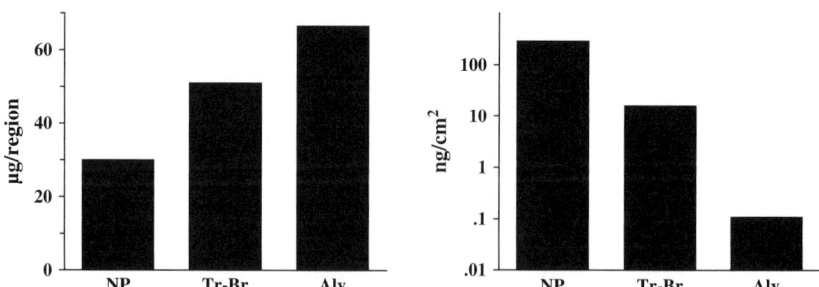

Fig. 1. Deposited dose per region (*left*) and surface area (*right*) in human nasopharyngeal (NP), tracheobronchial (Tr-Br), and alveolar (Alv) regions of the lung after inhalation of a polydisperse aerosol at 100 μg/m^3 with CMD 20 nm for 6 hours (MPPD). (*From* Oberdörster G. Kinetics of inhaled ultrafine particles in the organism. In: Heinrich U, editor. Effects of air contaminants on the respiratory tract: interpretations from molecular to meta analysis. 9th International Inhalation Symposium Monographs. Stuttgart (Germany): Fraunhofer IRB Verlag; 2004. p. 121; with permission.)

numerous as compared with coarse particles [26]. One might expect the regional number deposited dose to resemble the left half of Fig. 1.

This section focuses on the clearance of inhaled solid particles under non-overload conditions. By definition, lung particle overload results in the dysfunction of macrophage-mediated clearance, such that contact of inhaled material with the epithelium is likely, resulting in severe inflammation and translocation of particles to the interstitium and lung-associated lymph nodes. The clearance of deposited particles in the respiratory tract is basically governed by two processes: physical translocation of particles and chemical dissolution. The latter mechanism pertains to biosoluble particles or their components that are either lipid soluble or soluble in intracellular and extracellular fluids. Soluble components can then undergo absorption and diffusion or binding to proteins and other subcellular structures and eventually may be cleared into blood and lymphatic circulation. This mechanism of clearance for biosoluble materials can happen at any location within the respiratory tract. In contrast, there are several physical translocation processes, depending on the region in question.

The nasal mucosal and tracheobronchial regions combine the action of ciliated epithelial cells and a coating of mucous to form a mucociliary escalator that rapidly (approximately 24 hours) moves particles to the oropharynx, where they are swallowed into the gastrointestinal tract [27]. This clearance mechanism is likely to remove deposited UFP [28], although prolonged retention in the tracheobronchial region has been described [29]. In the alveolar region, the most prevalent clearance mechanism for deposited particles is phagocytosis by alveolar macrophages. Phagocytosis is facilitated by C5a, which attracts macrophages to the site of deposition [30]. The particle-laden macrophages migrate along the airways until they reach the mucociliary escalator, after which they are swallowed. Although the retention half-time of particles deposited in the alveolar region is several days (approximately 70 days in rodents; up to 700 days in humans [31]), most of them are phagocytosed by macrophages within the first 6 to 12 hours if they are of the optimal size.

Available data show that UFP are inefficiently cleared by alveolar macrophages; the optimal particle size for phagocytosis is 1 to 3 μm [23]. Fig. 2 displays results of studies in which rats were exposed to different types of particles of different sizes. Within 24 hours, approximately 80% of the 0.5-, 3-, and 10-μm particles could be retrieved in the macrophages fraction by extensive lung lavage, whereas only approximately 20% of ultrafine 15- to 20-nm and 80-nm particles could be lavaged with the macrophages. Conversely, approximately 80% of the UFP were retained in the lavaged lung after exhaustive lavage, and only approximately 20% of the larger particles remained in the lavaged lung. Recent results by Takenaka and coworkers [32] using inhaled 15-nm gold particles confirmed the inefficient uptake of UFP by macrophages. Because the lavage process reaches only the epithelial surface, it is likely that the UFP were taken up by epithelial cells or moved

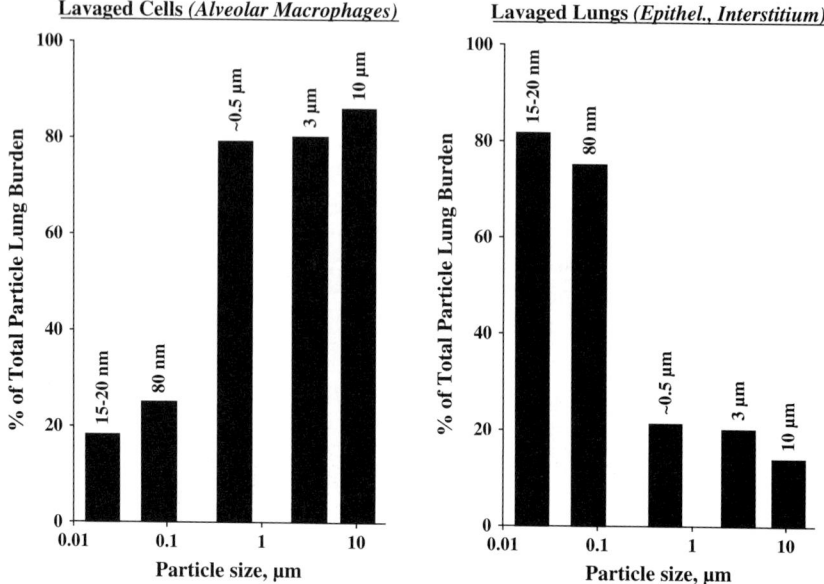

Fig. 2. Retention of ultrafine, fine, and coarse particles in rat alveolar macrophages 24 hours after exposure. (*From* Oberdörster G. Kinetics of inhaled ultrafine particles in the organism. In: Heinrich U, editor. Effects of air contaminants on the respiratory tract: interpretations from molecular to meta analysis. 9th International Inhalation Symposium Monographs. Stuttgart (Germany): Fraunhofer IRB Verlag; 2004. p. 121; with permission.)

into the interstitium. Several parallel or sequential events that determine the fate of deposited UFP can be envisioned: (1) uptake by epithelial cells (endocytosis, transcytosis); (2) movement between epithelial cells (tight junctions), thus being taken up by interstitial and endothelial cells; and (3) migration into blood and lymph circulation (Fig. 3). A combination of these processes is likely.

Several studies have been conducted to examine the accessibility of UFP deposited in the respiratory tract to epithelial and interstitial sites. For example, the fluorine-containing ultrafine particulate fraction in polytetrafluoroethylene fumes could be found in interstitial and submucosal sites of the conducting airways and in the interstitium of the periphery shortly after a 15-minute exposure [33]. The translocation process, however, seems to depend on particle size. In a study conducted in rats, more than 50% of a high dose of intratracheally instilled ultrafine TiO_2 (12 nm) translocated to the interstitium, whereas $\leq 4\%$ of fine TiO_2 (220 nm, 250 nm) translocated [34]. In general, interstitial translocation of fine particles across the alveolar epithelium is more prominent in larger species (dogs, nonhuman primates) than in rodents [27,35], so one may assume that the UFP translocation observed in rats also is likely to occur in humans. Experimental results in humans differ, however. One group reported the appearance in the liver of

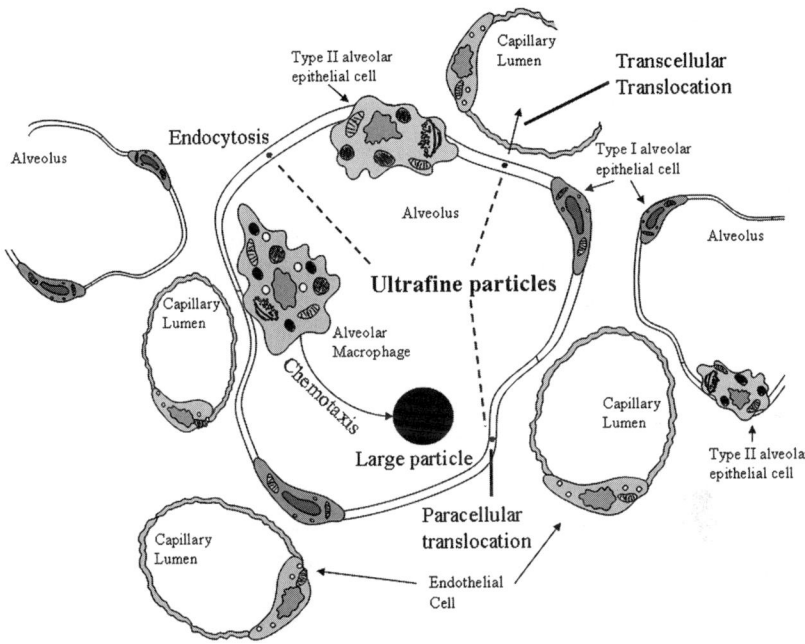

Fig. 3. Ultrastructure of pulmonary alveoli and capillaries showing potential routes of translocation of ultrafine, or nano-, particles out of the lungs.

a radiolabel attached to inhaled carbon UFP [36], but another study did not confirm this [37].

Once the particles have reached pulmonary interstitial sites, uptake into the blood and lymphatic circulation can occur. Studies in rats have shown that elemental ^{13}C UFP (count median diameter approximately 30 nm) accumulated to a large degree in the liver of rats within 24 hours after exposure, which indicated efficient translocation into the blood circulation [38]. Because rats were exposed via whole-body inhalation, the contribution to the signal from gastrointestinal tract exposure is difficult to separate from actual UFP translocation into the blood across the alveolar epithelium. Kreyling and colleagues [28] found only minimal translocation (<1%) from the lung to extrapulmonary organs in rats exposed to ^{192}Ir UFP via intratracheal inhalation; however, they reported tenfold greater translocation of 15-nm compared with 80-nm UFP. The conclusion from these studies is that translocation of inhaled UFP from the respiratory tract into the blood circulation can occur, possibly via mechanisms involving caveolae (transcytosis) that are present in alveolar epithelial and endothelial cell membranes [39,40]. The efficiency of the process may depend on UFP characteristics and the status of the lung epithelium, as suggested by studies using a rabbit model of acute lung injury induced by lipopolysaccharide [41].

The preceding sections focused on transcytosis and epithelial cellular uptake. Another fate must be considered, however, for particles that deposit in the respiratory tract, namely uptake by the sensory neuronal axons that are present in the nasopharyngeal, laryngeal, tracheobronchial, and alveolar regions of the lung [42]. Studies in rats have shown the transport of dye particles and microsphere tracers into trigeminal, nodose, and jugular ganglia after intratracheal and intranasal instillations [43,44]. Similarly, early studies showed that intranasally instilled 30-nm polio virus particles traveled along monkey olfactory nerve axons into the olfactory bulb [45,46]. Colloidal gold nanoparticles (50 nm) also have been shown to travel in the axon of olfactory nerves into the olfactory bulb of monkeys after intranasal instillations [47]. Both groups reported transport velocities of approximately 2.5 mm/h, which agrees well with axonal transport velocities after direct microinjection [48]. In a recent study, we found that inhalation of ^{13}C UFP (35 nm) by rats resulted in their significant accumulation in the olfactory bulb over a 7-day recovery period [49]. Results of another study in which rats were exposed to inhaled poorly soluble manganese oxide UFP (30 nm) for 11 days also showed significant increases of manganese in the olfactory bulb and the striatum, frontal cortex, and cerebellum [50]. These studies demonstrate that the olfactory nerve translocation route is also operable in rats for inhaled UFP deposited in the nasal region. This is not insignificant, considering that 5 to 20 nm particles deposit with equal efficiency in all regions of the respiratory tract, including the nose, and that UFP deposit at high numbers compared with larger particles.

Consequences of ultrafine particle translocation to extrapulmonary sites

We have discussed several mechanisms by which solid particles in the ultrafine and nano-sized range can gain access to extrapulmonary tissues, either by "escaping" the alveolo-capillary barrier or via neuronal translocation. The appearance of inhaled particles in the blood circulation could have several consequences. Studies by Nemmar and colleagues [15,16] demonstrated thrombogenic effects shortly after intravenous and intratracheal administration of positively charged polystyrene UFP and intratracheal diesel exhaust particles. The authors suggested that the responses were caused by the translocation of UFP from the alveolar region to the blood. Negatively charged and larger polystyrene particles were not thrombogenic in the hamster femoral vein model used. Using a similar model in rat ear veins, Silva and colleagues [51] showed the thrombogenic potential of elemental carbon UFP that were delivered via either intravenous injection or inhalation. It was hypothesized that UFP depositing in the alveoli are taken up by blood platelets after translocation from the alveoli, as shown with colloidal gold nanoparticles by Berry and colleagues [52], which results in their activation and thrombus formation with activated (primed) endothelial cells. The effects of PM on blood coagulation are reviewed in more detail in the article by Nemmar and colleagues in this issue. UFP that traverse the alveolo-capillary barrier conceivably could interact with or be taken up by endothelial cells, platelets, and leukocytes, potentially activating or injuring those cells. That activation/interaction could lead to endothelial dysfunction (eg, CD40, adhesion molecule upregulation; inflammatory cytokine upregulation; microparticle formation), coagulability, and thrombus formation and possibly lead to cardiac events. This sequence of events provides one potential mechanistic explanation for the adverse cardiovascular effects associated with environmental PM exposure in susceptible individuals. Our previous work with rats exposed to inhaled model UFP has shown changes in fibrinogen (suggesting changes in coagulability), endothelin-2 (suggesting vascular endothelial cell activation), thrombin-antithrombin complexes (indicative of thrombin generation), and the surface expression of intercellular adhesion molecule-1 on circulating neutrophils [18,19].

An area that has received a great deal of attention in recent years is the effect observed in epidemiologic, clinical, and animal studies of inhaled PM on the heart, which manifests in changes in heart rate and heart rate variability (HRV). For example, decreases in heart rate were found in humans exposed to inhaled fine- or ultrafine ambient PM [53,54]. Several studies also have shown decreases in time- and frequency-domain parameters of HRV with increases in ambient particulate air pollution [55–57]. In a clinical study, Frampton and associates [58] reported that exposures to laboratory-generated UFP caused a slight decrease in high frequency power (parasympathetic tone) during recovery from exercise immediately after exposure in healthy individuals. In an extensive, multicenter epidemiologic study on the effects of PM on HRV, investigators found that ultrafine—and not fine—particles were associated with decreases in vagosympathetic balance [59]. Using a rat model of surgically induced myocardial infarction, Wellenius and colleagues [60] reported that exposure to residual oil fly ash particles induced premature ventricular contractions and decreased overall HRV. We also reported a time-dependent decline in heart rate and vagosympathetic balance in telemetered hypertensive rats after exposure to freshly generated highway aerosols [61]. Several investigators have proposed that changes in HRV are predictive of arrhythmia (bradyarrhythmia or tachyarrhythmia) and poor outcome after exposure to PM in individuals with compromised cardiovascular systems [62,63]. The cardiovascular effects of PM are reviewed in more detail in the article by Godleski in this issue.

The concept that the central nervous system could be a potential target for inhaled solid particles is an intriguing one. Because of an accelerated onset of parkinsonism in welders [64] and the high levels of manganese in welding fumes [65–67], many studies have focused on the accumulation and effects of manganese in the brain. Studies conducted in rats have shown translocation of soluble manganese compounds along olfactory neuronal pathways to the olfactory bulb after inhalation or intranasal instillation exposures [68–70]. We also observed an increase in olfactory bulb manganese after ultrafine manganese oxide inhalation exposure [50]. Although Henriksson and Tjälve [69] found changes in markers of astrocyte activation (eg, glial flibrillary acidic protein) in several brain regions from rats exposed intranasally to soluble manganese chloride, Dorman and colleagues [68] did not find these changes after exposure to manganese sulfate or phosphate. Factors potentially contributing to the lack of concurrence in results include differences in the solubilities of the manganese salts used, the doses, and the contribution of olfactory epithelial damage in some cases. In a series of studies using postmortem brain tissues from canines and humans living in Mexico City, Calderón-Garcidueñas and coworkers [71–73] showed inflammatory mediator production, blood-brain barrier disruption, cell degeneration, and DNA damage in the cortex, hippocampus, and olfactory bulb associated with exposure to high levels of air pollution. Although ultrafine and other particulate levels were not directly assessed as part of these studies and the ambient pollutant mixture also contains numerous oxidant gases and metals, the findings suggest that the central nervous system is a target for real-world particulate-containing aerosols. Using two distinct size fractions of concentrated fine PM from a roadside ($PM_{2.5}$, PM < 180 nm), Campbell and colleagues [74] showed inflammatory changes in cortical neurons from mouse brain after concentrated PM exposure. Although the two size fractions were large compared with the peak of the ultrafine mode in ambient air, UFP would be included in both.

Summary

Several conclusions can be drawn from this brief review of the concepts related to ultrafine and nano-particle disposition and effects. One critical point is that particles in the ultrafine or nano-size range have high deposition efficiency throughout the respiratory tract. Second, several studies have shown their translocation to extrapulmonary sites via the circulation under certain conditions. Transport via sensory nerves to the central nervous system also seems to occur. Based on animal studies, the consequences of UFP exposure include inflammation and oxidative stress at the site of deposition or translocation. Effects are not limited to the lung, the portal of entry, but also have been found in the cardiovascular and central nervous systems. It is apparent from the existing studies that translocation of and responses to UFP depend on dose, chemistry, surface area or shape, length of exposure, and the general health of the exposed individual. A clear definition of the extent to which these variables affect biologic responses is the subject of ongoing research.

References

[1] Schwartz J, Dockery DW. Increased mortality in Philadelphia associated with daily air pollution concentrations. Am Rev Respir Dis 1992;145:600–4.

[2] Peters A, Wichmann H-E, Tuch T, et al. Respiratory effects are associated with the number of ultrafine particles. Am J Respir Crit Care Med 1997;155:1376–83.

[3] Peters A, von Klot S, Heier M, et al. Exposure to traffic and the onset of myocardial infarction. N Engl J Med 2004;351(17):1721–30.

[4] Pope CA III. Epidemiology of fine particulate air pollution and human health: biologic mechanisms and who's at risk? Environ Health Perspect 2000;108(Suppl 4):713–23.

[5] Wichmann H-E, Spix C, Tuch T, et al. Daily mortality and fine and ultrafine particles in Erfurt, Germany. Part I. Role of particle number and particle mass. Res Rep Health Eff Inst 2000;98:5–86.

[6] Pekkanen J, Peters A, Hoek G, et al. Particulate air pollution and risk of ST-segment depression during repeated submaximal exercise tests among subjects with coronary heart disease: the exposure and risk assessment for fine and ultrafine particles in ambient air (ULTRA) study. Circulation 2002;106(8):933–8.

[7] Zanobetti A, Schwartz J. Are diabetics more susceptible to the health effects of airborne particles? Am J Respir Crit Care Med 2001;164(5):831–3.

[8] Frampton MW, Utell MJ, Zareba W, et al. Effects of exposure to ultrafine carbon particles in healthy subjects and subjects with asthma. Res Rep Health Eff Inst 2004;126:1–47.

[9] Frampton MW, Stewart JC, Oberdörster G, et al. Inhalation of ultrafine particles alters blood leukocyte expression of adhesion molecules in humans. Environ Health Perspect 2006;114(1):51–8.

[10] Li XY, Gilmour PS, Donaldson K, et al. Free radical activity and pro-inflammatory effects of particulate air pollution (PM_{10}) in vivo and in vitro. Thorax 1996;51:1216–22.

[11] Elder ACP, Gelein R, Finkelstein JN, et al. The pulmonary inflammatory response to inhaled ultrafine particles is modified by age, ozone exposure, and bacterial toxin. Inhal Toxicol 2000;12:227–46.

[12] Elder ACP, Carter J, Corson N, et al. Endotoxin priming, ozone exposure, and age affect ultrafine particle-induced inflammation and antioxidant gene expression in mouse lung and heart. Am J Respir Crit Care Med 2002;165(8):A537.

[13] Elder A, Corson N, Gelein R, et al. Influenza virus, ozone exposure, and age modify the inflammatory response to ultrafine particles in mouse lung. Am J Respir Crit Care Med 2003; 167(7):A761.

[14] Zhou YM, Zhong CY, Kennedy IM, et al. Pulmonary responses of acute exposure to ultrafine iron particles in healthy adult rats. Environ Toxicol 2003;18(4):227–35.

[15] Nemmar A, Hoylaerts M, Hoet PHM, et al. Ultrafine particles affect experimental thrombosis in an in vivo hamster model. Am J Respir Crit Care Med 2002;166:998–1004.

[16] Nemmar A, Nemery B, Hoet PH, et al. Pulmonary inflammation and thrombogenicity caused by diesel particles in hamsters: role of histamine. Am J Respir Crit Care Med 2003; 168:1366–72.

[17] Wellenius GA, Coull BA, Godleski JJ, et al. Inhalation of concentrated ambient air particles exacerbates myocardial ischemia in conscious dogs. Environ Health Perspect 2003;111: 402–8.

[18] Elder ACP, Gelein R, Azadniv M, et al. Systemic effects of inhaled ultrafine particles in two compromised, aged rat strains. Inhal Toxicol 2004;16:461–71.

[19] Elder A, Gelein R, Finkelstein J, et al. On-road exposure to highway aerosols: II. Exposures of aged, compromised rats. Inhal Toxicol 2004;16:41–53.

[20] Sun Q, Wang A, Jin X, et al. Long-term air pollution exposure and acceleration of atherosclerosis and vascular inflammation in an animal model. JAMA 2005;294:3003–10.

[21] US Environmental Protection Agency. Air quality criteria for particulate matter. Research Triangle Park (NC): National Center for Environmental Assessment-RTP Office; 2004. Report No. EPA /600/P-99/002aF-bF.2v.

[22] International Commission on Radiological Protection. Human respiratory tract model for radiological protection: a report of committee 2 of the ICRP. Oxford: Pergamon Press; 1994.

[23] Hahn FF, Newton GJ, Bryant PL. *In vitro* phagocytosis of respirable-sized monodisperse particles by alveolar macrophages. In: Sanders CL, Schneider RP, Dagle GE, et al, editors. Pulmonary macrophages and epithelial cells (ERDA Series 43). Oak Ridge (TN): Technical Information Center, Energy Research and Development Administration; 1977. p. 424–35.

[24] Oberdörster G. Kinetics of inhaled ultrafine particles in the organism. In: Heinrich U, editor. Effects of air contaminants on the respiratory tract: interpretations from molecular to meta analysis (9th INIS Monographs). Stuttgart (Germany): Fraunhofer IRB Verlag; 2004. p. 121.

[25] Asgharian B, Anjilvel S. A multi-path model of fiber deposition in the rat lung. Toxicol Sci 1998;44:80–6.

[26] Pekkanen J, Timonen KL, Ruuskanen J, et al. Effects of ultrafine and fine particles in urban air on peak expiratory flow among children with asthmatic symptoms. Environ Res 1997;74: 24–33.

[27] Kreyling W, Scheuch G. Clearance of particles deposited in the lungs. In: Gehr P, Heyder J, editors. Particle-lung interactions. New York: Marcel Dekker; 2000. p. 323–76.

[28] Kreyling WG, Semmler M, Erbe F, et al. Ultrafine insoluble iridium particles are negligibly translocated from lung epithelium to extrapulmonary organs. J Toxicol Environ Health 2002;65(20):1513–30.

[29] Stahlhofen W, Scheuch G, Bailey MR. Investigations of retention of inhaled particles in the human bronchial tree. Radiat Prot Dosimetry 1995;60(4):311–9.

[30] Warheit DB, Overby LH, George G, et al. Pulmonary macrophages are attracted to inhaled particles on alveolar surfaces. Exp Lung Res 1988;14:51–66.

[31] Kreyling WG. Interspecies comparison of lung clearance of "insoluble" particles. J Aerosol Med 1990;3F:S93–110.

[32] Takenaka S, Karg E, Kreyling WG, et al. Distribution pattern of inhaled ultrafine gold particles in the rat lung. Inhal Toxicol 2006;18(10):733–40.

[33] Oberdörster G, Finkelstein JN, Johnston C, et al. Acute pulmonary effects of ultrafine particles in rats and mice. Res Rep Health Eff Inst 2000;96:1–74.

[34] Oberdörster G, Ferin J, Gelein R, et al. Role of the alveolar macrophage in lung injury: studies with ultrafine particles. Environ Health Perspect 1992;97:193–7.

[35] Nikula KJ, Avila KJ, Griffith WC, et al. Lung tissue responses and sites of particle retention differ between rats and Cynomolgus monkeys exposed chronically to diesel exhaust and coal dust. Fundam Appl Toxicol 1997;37:37–53.

[36] Nemmar A, Hoet PHM, Vanquickenborne B, et al. Passage of inhaled particles into the blood circulation in humans. Circulation 2002;105:411–4.

[37] Wiebert P, Sanchez-Crespo A, Falk R, et al. No significant translocation of inhaled 35-nm carbon particles to the circulation in humans. Inhal Toxicol 2006;18(10):741–7.

[38] Oberdörster G, Sharp Z, Atudorei V, et al. Extrapulmonary translocation of ultrafine carbon particles following whole-body inhalation exposure of rats. J Toxicol Environ Health 2002;65:1531–43.

[39] Gumbleton M. Caveolae as potential macromolecule trafficking compartments within alveolar epithelium. Adv Drug Deliv Rev 2001;49:281–300.

[40] Mehta D, Bhattacharya J, Matthay MA, et al. Integrated control of lung fluid balance. Am J Physiol 2004;287:L1081–90.

[41] Heckel K, Kiefmann R, Dörger M, et al. Colloidal gold particles as a new in vivo marker of early acute lung injury. Am J Physiol 2006;287:L867–78.

[42] Yeates DB. Neurally mediated cardiopulmonary and systemic responses to inhaled irritants and antigens. In: Gehr P, Heyder J, editors. Particle-lung interactions. New York: Marcel Dekker; 2000. p. 603–26.

[43] Hunter DD, Dey RD. Identification and neuropeptide content of trigeminal neurons innervating the rat nasal epithelium. Neuroscience 1998;83(2):591–9.

[44] Hunter DD, Undem BJ. Identification of substance P content of vagal afferent neurons innervating the epithelium of the guinea pig trachea. Am J Respir Crit Care Med 1999;159: 1943–8.

[45] Bodian D, Howe HA. The rate of progression of poliomyelitis virus in nerves. Bull Johns Hopkins Hosp 1941;69(No. 2):79–85.

[46] Howe HA, Bodian D. Poliomyelitis in the chimpanzee: a clinical-pathological study. Bull Johns Hopkins Hosp 1941;69(No. 2):149–82.

[47] DeLorenzo AJD. The olfactory neuron and the blood-brain barrier. In: Wolstenholme GEW, Knight J, editors. Taste and smell in vertebrates. London: J&A Churchill; 1970. p. 151–76.

[48] Adams RJ, Bray D. Rapid transport of foreign particles microinjected into crab axons. Nature 1983;303:718–20.

[49] Oberdörster G, Sharp Z, Atudorei V, et al. Translocation of inhaled ultrafine particles to the brain. Inhal Toxicol 2004;16:437–45.

[50] Elder AR, Gelein V, Silva V, et al. Translocation of inhaled ultrafine manganese oxide particles to the central nervous system. Environ Health Perspect 2006;114(8)1172–8.

[51] Silva VM, Corson N, Elder A, et al. The rat ear vein model for investigating in vivo thrombogenicity of ultrafine particles (UFP). Toxicol Sci 2005;85:983–9.

[52] Berry JP, Arnoux B, Stanislas G, et al. A microanalytic study of particles transport across the alveoli: role of blood platelets. Biomedicine 1977;27:354–7.

[53] Gold DR, Litonjua A, Schwartz J, et al. Ambient pollution and heart rate variability. Circulation 2000;101:1267–73.

[54] Ibald-Mulli A, Timonen KL, Peters A, et al. Effects of particulate air pollution on blood pressure and heart rate in subjects with cardiovascular disease: a multicenter approach. Environ Health Perspect 2004;112:369–77.

[55] Creason J, Neas L, Walsh D, et al. Particulate matter and heart rate variability among elderly retirees: the Baltimore 1998 PM study. J Expo Anal Environ Epidemiol 2001;11(2):116–22.

[56] Devlin RB, Ghio AJ, Kehrl H, et al. Elderly humans exposed to concentrated air pollution particles have decreased heart rate variability. Eur Respir J Suppl 2003;40:76s–80s.

[57] Holguin F, Tellez-Rojo MM, Hernandez M, et al. Air pollution and heart rate variability among the elderly in Mexico City. Epidemiology 2003;14(5):521–7.

[58] Frampton MW, Zareba W, Daigle CC, et al. Inhalation of ultrafine particles alters myocardial repolarization in humans. Am J Respir Crit Care Med 2002;165(8):B16.

[59] Timonen KL, Vanninen E, de Hartog J, et al. Effects of ultrafine and fine particulate and gaseous air pollution on cardiac autonomic control in subjects with coronary artery disease: the ULTRA study. J Expo Anal Environ Epidemiol 2006;16(4):332–41.

[60] Wellenius GA, Saldiva PHN, Batalha JRF, et al. Electrocardiographic changes during exposure to residual oil fly ash (ROFA) particles in a rat model of myocardial infarction. Toxicol Sci 2002;66:327–35.

[61] Elder ACP, Couderc J-P, Corson N, et al. Autonomic responses to inhaled on-road highway aerosols in telemetered spontaneously hypertensive rats. Inhal Toxicol 2006; in press.

[62] Tsuji H, Larson MG, Vendetti FJ Jr, et al. Impact of reduced heart rate variability on risk of cardiac events: the Framingham heart study. Circulation 1996;94:2850–5.

[63] Stone PH, Godleski JJ. First steps toward understanding the pathophysiologic link between air pollution and cardiac mortality. Am Heart J 1999;138:804–7.

[64] Racette BA, McGee-Minnich L, Moerlein SM, et al. Welding-related parkinsonism: clinical features, treatment, and pathophysiology. Neurol 2001;56(1):8–13.

[65] Korczynski RE. Occupational health concerns in the welding industry. Appl Occup Environ Hyg 2000;15(12):936–45.

[66] Li GJ, Zhang LL, Lu L, et al. Occupational exposure to welding fume among welders: alterations of manganese, iron, zinc, copper, and lead in body fluids and the oxidative stress status. J Occup Environ Med 2004;46(3):241–8.

[67] Sinczuk-Walczak H, Jacubowski M, Matczak W. Neurological and neurophysiological examinations of workers occupationally exposed to manganese. Int J Occup Med Environ Health 2001;14(4):329–37.

[68] Dorman DC, McManus BE, Parkinson CU, et al. Nasal toxicity of manganese sulfate and manganese phosphate in young male rats following subchronic (13-week) inhalation exposure. Inhal Toxicol 2004;16(6–7):481–8.

[69] Henricksson J, Tjälve H. Manganese taken up into the CNS via the olfactory pathway in rats affects astrocytes. Toxicol Sci 2000;55:392–8.

[70] Tjälve H, Henricksson J. Uptake of metals in the brain via olfactory pathways. Neurotoxicol 1999;20:181–96.

[71] Calderón-Garcidueñas L, Azzarelli B, Acuna H, et al. Air pollution and brain damage. Toxicol Pathol 2002;30(3):373–89.

[72] Calderón-Garcidueñas L, Maronpot RR, Torres-Jardon R, et al. DNA damage in nasal and brain tissues of canines exposed to air pollutants is associated with evidence of chronic brain inflammation and neurodegeneration. Toxicol Pathol 2003;31(5):524–38.

[73] Calderón-Garcidueñas L, Reed W, Maronpot RR, et al. Brain inflammation and Alzheimer's-like pathology in individuals exposed to severe air pollution. Toxicol Pathol 2004;32(6):650–8.

[74] Campbell A, Oldham M, Becaria A, et al. Particulate matter in polluted air may increase biomarkers of inflammation in mouse brain. Neurotoxicology 2005;26:133–40.

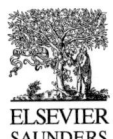

ELSEVIER
SAUNDERS

Clin Occup Environ Med
5 (4) 797–815

CLINICS IN
OCCUPATIONAL AND
ENVIRONMENTAL
MEDICINE

Inflammation and Airborne Particles

Mark W. Frampton, MD

*Division of Pulmonary and Critical Care Medicine, University of Rochester Medical Center,
601 Elmwood Avenue, Rochester, NY 14642-8692, USA*

Inflammation provides a potential mechanistic link between inhalation of particles and the diverse health effects found in epidemiologic studies. Considerable uncertainty remains as to the importance of inflammation in mediating these effects and where that inflammation is occurring: lung, vascular endothelium, or distant organs, including the heart. This article briefly reviews the role of inflammation in pulmonary and cardiovascular disease and explores the evidence that the health effects of particulate matter (PM) exposure are mediated, at least in part, by inflammation.

Inflammation as a disease process

The clinical characteristics that define inflammation are well known to anyone who has suffered from a soft tissue infection or injury. The first clinical description has been attributed the Roman physician, Cornelius Celsus: dolor (pain), rubor (redness), tumor (swelling), and calor (heat). Virchow subsequently added an additional feature, functio laesa, or loss of function [1]. There are three primary features: vascular changes, migration and activation of leukocytes, and systemic reactions.

In acute inflammation, vascular dilatation and increased blood flow increase delivery of leukocytes to the affected region, and increased vascular permeability allows movement of plasma proteins into the affected tissues. Vascular endothelium and blood leukocytes display surface selectins and integrins that lead to slowing, rolling, attachment, and migration of leukocytes into the affected tissue. These processes are tightly orchestrated by various locally released chemokines and other mediators. Scientific progress over the last decade has shed light on the cellular and signaling mechanisms that control the inflammatory responses. Inflammation is intertwined with

This work was supported by grants RO1 ES011853, RO1 ES013394, RR00044, and ES01247 from the National Institutes of Health.

E-mail address: mark_frampton@urmc.rochester.edu

doi:10.1016/j.coem.2006.07.006

the complement system and the coagulation cascade. These relationships are indicated schematically in Fig. 1.

The major purposes of inflammation are to defend the host against invading microorganisms and repair injury. Wherever there is injury there is inflammation, even in the absence of infection. Leukocytes are recruited to areas of injury. When these cells encounter bacterial lipopolysaccharide and peptides, the nicotinamide adenine dinucleotide phosphate (NADPH)-oxidase enzyme system is activated to release reactive oxygen species that kill bacteria. Leukocytes also release various proteolytic enzymes, in part to clear the "coagulum" and gain access to infected tissue and to kill the pathogen. They internalize pathogens and dead host tissue by phagocytosis. Activated macrophages and local dendritic cells process antigenic proteins from the internalized invading organism and present these protein fragments to lymphocytes along with costimulating molecules. This initiates specific cellular and humoral responses, with the goal of preventing successful invasion of the organism in the future. Many of the inflammatory products released by recruited leukocytes also damage healthy tissue.

Inflammation is a response to injury from causes other than infection. Whether the injury is from trauma or inhalation of a toxic air contaminant, debris from devitalized tissue must be cleared and healing initiated. The inflammatory cascade is a vital component of the response to injury and cell death. Vascular dilatation delivers inflammatory cells to clear debris and digest dead tissue, along with oxygen-carrying red blood cells and even progenitor cells. An exaggerated or persistent inflammatory response may cause loss of function through tissue remodeling and scarring, however.

In the case of exposure to environmental pollutants, including ambient PM, inflammation may represent a marker of cell and tissue injury from the exposure. Alternatively, PM or its chemical components may activate cellular host defense pathways, in a sense mimicking an infectious agent, with the subsequent inflammatory response causing cellular injury. In this

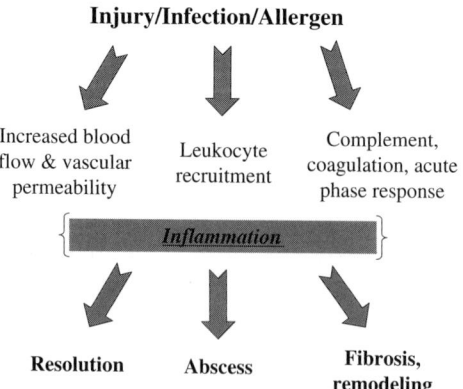

Fig. 1. Causes and effects of inflammation.

case, tissue injury is a consequence of the inflammatory response rather than its cause.

How is inflammation measured?

Table 1 shows some of the methods for assessing inflammation in human studies of the effects of PM exposure. Inflammation in any tissue can be measured directly by histologic examination, the gold standard, which allows quantitation of inflammatory cells, vascularity, cell injury, and necrosis. This generally requires an invasive procedure in the human subject or sacrifice of the experimental animal, however. Airway epithelium can be sampled in humans using bronchoscopy and bronchial biopsy, but this entails discomfort and some risk. Airway inflammation can be assessed by recovery of inflammatory cells from bronchoalveolar lavage fluid or induced

Table 1
Methods for assessing inflammation

Method	Advantages	Disadvantages
Spirometry (FEV$_1$)	Noninvasive, standardized, reproducible, correlated with functional status	Not sensitive or specific for inflammation
Nonspecific airways responsiveness	Noninvasive, somewhat standardized	Not well correlated with airway inflammation; relatively time consuming and expensive
Exhaled breath nitric oxide	Noninvasive, method standardized	Influenced by factors other than inflammation; lacks sensitivity
Exhaled breath condensate	Noninvasive	Limited to inflammatory mediators and products (no cells), variable dilution limits quantitation
Plasma acute phase proteins	Minimally invasive	Nonspecific; reflects general inflammatory burden, influenced by nutrition and general health
Plasma Clara cell protein	Minimally invasive, marker of lung epithelial permeability	Not specific for inflammation, may lack sensitivity, functional significance unclear
Induced sputum	Noninvasive, inexpensive	Unpleasant for subject, may induce bronchoconstriction in people with asthma; samples only large airways
Airway appearance	Reflects multiple aspects of inflammation	Invasive (requires bronchoscopy), lacks sensitivity and specificity
Airway lavage	Cell recovery often reflects tissue inflammation, less invasive than biopsy	Invasive (requires bronchoscopy); findings vary with methodology; samples airway cells; may not accurately reflect tissue events
Histology	The "gold standard"; direct measure of inflammatory cells	Invasive; samples often small, may not be representative

sputum. Exhaled nitric oxide and carbon monoxide and measurements in exhaled breath condensate are promising methods for measuring the products of inflammatory processes, but they lack sensitivity and specificity. Cardiac and vascular inflammation is more difficult to assess directly in the living animal or human.

Soluble markers of inflammation that can be measured in blood or body fluids include inflammatory cytokine gene or protein expression. Indirect measures of airway inflammation include decrements in pulmonary function secondary to airway narrowing, increases in nonspecific airways responsiveness, and increases in plasma markers of systemic inflammation, such as c-reactive protein or fibrinogen.

In general, the less invasive methods for assessing airway inflammation also suffer from reduced sensitivity or specificity. For example, FEV_1 may decrease in people with asthma when airway inflammation worsens. In healthy people, however, considerable inflammation may be present without impairment in FEV_1. Lung function decrements may occur via mechanisms that differ from the inflammatory pathways, as has been shown for exposure to ozone [2].

The genetics of inflammation

The complexity and diversity of inflammatory pathways involve many genes, with many opportunities for differences among individuals in the nature and intensity of the inflammatory response. It is likely that susceptibility to the health effects of PM exposure are genetically influenced in healthy individuals and persons who have asthma [3]. For example, in human volunteers with ragweed allergy, nasal instillation of diesel exhaust particles (DEP) enhanced local IgE production in response to ragweed allergen to a greater degree in subjects with the glutathione-S-transferase M1 null genotype than in subjects with the functional genotype [4]. Studies in animals and healthy humans of the responses to lipopolysaccharide—the cell membrane component of gram-negative bacteria that initiates fever and sepsis—has helped to define some of the genetic determinants of variability in the innate immune responses [5]. Approximately 3000 to 5000 genes, up to 20% of the human genome, are involved in the healthy inflammatory response to lipopolysaccharide [6]. Gene expression profiling studies are attempting to define unique patterns of gene expression for specific clinical scenarios involving inflammation [7]. It is hoped that these same approaches will provide gene expression profiles specific for air pollution exposures and sources.

Inflammation and pulmonary disease

There is evidence that inhalation of outdoor air particles can cause inflammation in the lungs. Ghio and colleagues [8] exposed healthy volunteers to concentrated ambient fine particles (CAPs) in Chapel Hill, NC. Bronchoscopy with bronchoalveolar lavage demonstrated a modest increase in the recovery of neutrophils compared with clean air exposure (Fig. 2), similar to what has been observed after exposure to ozone. In contrast, in a different laboratory, inhalation of CAPs in Southern California caused no changes in inflammatory cells in induced sputum [9]. Pietropaoli and colleagues [10] exposed subjects to 10 to 25 $\mu g/m^3$ elemental carbon ultrafine particles (UFPs) for 2 hours, with intermittent exercise. They found no effects on sputum inflammatory cells, pulmonary function, or exhaled nitric oxide (NO), a noninvasive measure of airway inflammation. Additional studies at a higher concentration (50 $\mu g/m^3$) also showed no changes in pulmonary function or exhaled NO, and no changes were seen in systemic markers of inflammation or coagulation [11]. These studies suggest that inhalation of fine particles induces mild inflammation in the distal airways, which is sampled by bronchoalveolar lavage, but not proximal airways, which are sampled by induced sputum and exhaled NO. Whether inhalation of UFPs causes distal airway inflammation in humans has not been determined.

Animal studies also provide evidence that CAPs cause airway inflammation. Distal airway inflammation has been described in rats acutely exposed to concentrated ambient particles [12]. In a recently completed study of long-term exposure to concentrated ambient fine particles in mice [13], the only organ system that was examined that did not exhibit CAPs-related responses was the pulmonary system. There was no evidence for lung inflammation as indicated by lavage parameters (cell counts and protein levels) and histopathology. Because the lung is the portal of entry for the CAPs,

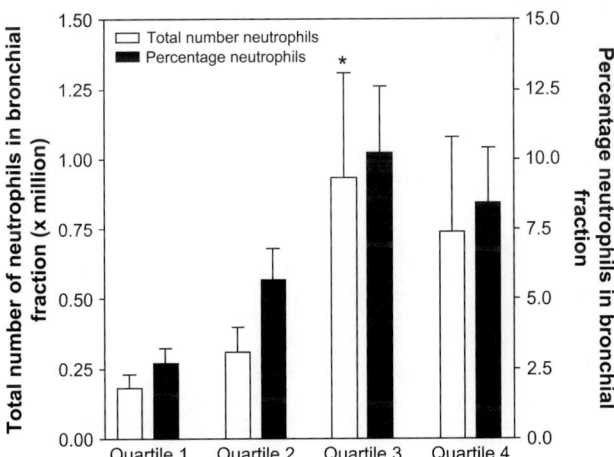

Fig. 2. Neutrophil numbers in the bronchial fraction after inhalation of particles and filtered air. The number and percentage of neutrophils in the bronchial fraction of the lavage increased with particle inhalation. (*From* Ghio AJ, Kim C, Devlin RB. Concentrated ambient air particles induce mild pulmonary inflammation in healthy human volunteers. Am J Respir Crit Care Med 2000;162:985; with permission from the American Thoracic Society. Copyright © 2000 American Thoracic Society.)

the investigators had anticipated that some changes would be observed in this organ system. Tolerance or adaptation to inflammation after repeated exposure to particles or gases has been reported in humans and animals. In this sense, it was not surprising that no persistent inflammatory change was observed after repeated exposure of low levels of CAPs in this study. Absence of persistent inflammation does not imply that there was no exposure-related reaction to CAPs in the lung, however. Subclinical change could have occurred that could not be detected by the measurement methods that were used in this study (ie, transient changes in the lung could have occurred and been resolved by the end of the 5-month exposure period). Lung cells (epithelia cells and macrophages) also could have been actively secreting cytokines or chemokines without inflammatory changes.

Although there is evidence that inhalation of ambient air particles causes distal airway inflammation acutely, it is unclear what role lung inflammation plays in the short- and long-term health effects of PM. It is less clear what role PM-induced airway inflammation plays in worsening respiratory disease. We explore these issues for asthma, chronic obstructive pulmonary disease (COPD), and smoking.

Asthma

Inflammation plays a critical role in the obstructive airway diseases—asthma and COPD. In asthma, airway inflammation is part of what defines the disease. Inflammation is present even in people with mild disease who do not have symptomatic bronchoconstriction.

The asthmatic airway is characterized by increased numbers of eosinophils, lymphocytes, and neutrophils, with destruction of the ciliated epithelium and remodeling of the subepithelial structures. The inflammatory processes are characterized as T-helper-2, in which lymphocytes and other inflammatory cells produce interleukin-4, -5, and -13, with recruitment of eosinophils into the airway mucosa. This T-helper-2 response, evolved to protect against parasitic infection, can make exposure to allergens dangerous. The asthmatic airway constricts when challenged with specific allergen and is hyperresponsive to nonspecific irritants and aerosols. Sulfur dioxide inhalation reproducibly constricts the airways of many people with asthma and has been used as a measure of airway responsiveness [14]. A complete review of inflammation in the pathogenesis of asthma is beyond the scope of this article but is available elsewhere [15,16]. The key question with regard to air pollution health effects is whether particulate air pollution causes or exacerbates airway inflammation in asthma.

There are several reasons why people who have asthma are considered at increased risk for adverse effects from ambient PM exposure. First, obstructive lung disease increases the airway deposition rate of fine particles and UFPs [17,18]. Second, the nonspecific airways responsiveness characteristic of asthma suggests that people who have asthma may respond to lower concentrations of irritant particles than healthy people. Third, if PM exposure further increases the underlying airway inflammation, it would be expected to worsen disease severity and would increase the airway responses to allergen exposure. For example, inhalation of ozone during exercise increases the recovery of inflammatory cells from the airways of healthy people [2] and people who have asthma [19] and enhances responsiveness to specific allergen challenge in individuals who have asthma [20,21].

There is abundant evidence from epidemiology studies that PM air pollution contributes to asthma exacerbations. Atmospheric particles, including acid aerosols derived from SO_2 emissions, have been linked with worsening of symptoms, decrements in lung function, increased hospital admissions for asthma, and increased medication use [22–24]. Studies in the early 1980s demonstrated that exposure to acid aerosols reduces pulmonary function in persons who have asthma [25]. The concentrations required to cause effects were considerably higher than ambient air concentrations, however.

Two studies found that exposure to acid aerosols, either followed by [26] or in combination with [27] ozone exposure, increased airway responsiveness to ozone in subjects who have asthma at concentrations of acid aerosol well below those known to cause changes in lung function or airway inflammation in the absence of ozone. This finding suggests that exposures to acid aerosols may enhance the airway effects of ozone or bring out effects at lower concentrations in people with asthma.

A recent study suggested that increases in ambient PM in the Seattle, Washington area associated with increased airway inflammation in children who have asthma, as determined by increased exhaled NO concentrations [28]. There is little evidence from clinical studies that exposure to ambient PM causes acute bronchoconstriction or worsens airway inflammation in asthma. For example, 2-hour exposures to concentrated ambient fine PM in the Los Angeles, California area did not reduce pulmonary function or increase sputum inflammatory cells in subjects who have mild asthma [9]. Similarly, 2-hour exposures to 10 $\mu g/m^3$ ultrafine elemental carbon particles did not alter lung function or sputum inflammatory cells in subjects who have asthma [10]. It is possible that children are more susceptible than adults, that Seattle PM causes more inflammation than Los Angeles PM, that the whole mixture of gaseous and particulate pollutants is necessary to cause inflammation, or that induced sputum lacks sufficient sensitivity. It is also possible that the increase in exhaled NO seen in Seattle was caused by something other than inflammation. Clearly, more work is needed to understand the role of inflammation in the relationship between PM and asthma.

Exposure to DEP may represent a special case with regard to asthma. This issue has been reviewed [29], and was the subject of a workshop [30]. There is suggestive evidence that certain kinds of PM exposure, such as DEP, may contribute to the cause of asthma in susceptible people.

Many published studies have shown positive associations between traffic density and respiratory symptoms and illness in children, including cough, wheeze, bronchitis, asthma, runny nose, allergic rhinitis, and decreased lung function [31–35]. Some studies have used proximity to the roadway, or truck counts, as surrogates for the intensity of DEP exposure. These studies have almost exclusively been in Europe and Japan, where the proportion of diesel vehicles is larger than in the United States. Associations are generally stronger with truck traffic density, and with ambient air markers of diesel exhaust (elemental carbon levels, particle number). These findings support, but do not prove, that DEP are a factor in causing these symptoms and illnesses. Many of these studies have attempted to control for potential sources of bias. However, it is difficult to completely exclude confounding factors that may be related to living near high traffic areas, such as differing socioeconomic status, tobacco smoke exposure, other pollution sources, differences in medical care, and quality of life influences. Furthermore, most of these studies address symptoms, but not clinical asthma.

Exposure to diesel exhaust at relatively high concentrations of 200-300 $\mu g/m^3$ for 1 hour, with intermittent exercise, caused airway inflammation in humans [36]. Neutrophils increased in bronchoalveolar lavage fluid, as well as expression of adhesion molecules and interleukin-8 in airway biopsy tissue [37]. In subjects with mild asthma, exposure to diesel exhaust at particle concentrations of 300 $\mu g/m^3$ for 1 hour increased airway resistance and hyperresponsiveness [38]. However, increases in inflammatory markers were not more intense than in healthy subjects.

Clinical studies provide evidence for the plausibility that DEP may contribute to allergen sensitization, and by implication, to causation of asthma. The nasal response to 300 μg resuspended DEP, administered by nasal spray, has been studied in both healthy and asthmatic subjects [39]. DEP induced an increase in nasal IgE, and in IgE-producing cells, in nasal lavage fluid. There was also increased production of both T_H1 and T_H2 cytokines by cells in the nasal lavage fluid [40]. In subjects with ragweed allergy, intranasal challenge with DEP and ragweed allergen markedly enhanced the production of ragweed-specific IgE (but not total IgE) compared with ragweed alone, and resulted in a decreased production of T_H1 cytokines and increased production of T-helper-2 and other cytokines [41]. The relevance of nasal instillation as a model for inhalation of ambient concentrations of diesel is not established, and the effect of DEP on lower airway allergic responses has not been studied. Furthermore, the effects could represent non-specific particle responses, because other types of particles were not studied. Nevertheless, these studies provide evidence that DEP enhance allergic responses in the human airway mucosa, a possible mechanism for induction of allergic asthma.

Chronic obstructive pulmonary disease

The term COPD encompasses various pathophysiologic states associated with obstruction to air flow. The obstruction is relatively fixed, which differentiates this condition from asthma, in which reversibility or variability in airflow obstruction is a cardinal feature. Inflammation and narrowing of the airways and loss of lung parenchyma and elastic tissue contribute to the collapse of small airways during expiration. Three main pathophysiologic elements are seen in patients with COPD: chronic bronchitis, emphysema or acinar enlargement, and narrowing of small, distal airways [42]. For a given patient, the relative involvement with these three types of pathology determines in part the symptoms, signs, and course of COPD. The pathophysiology of these disease types may confer different susceptibilities to the effects of air pollutant exposure. For example, patients who have COPD may have predominantly chronic bronchitis, with cough, sputum production, and failure of the right side of the heart, or emphysema, with more severe shortness of breath but less cough and sputum production. It is likely that persons with these disease subsets differ in their susceptibility to the effects of particle exposure.

Inflammation is present in the lungs of patients who have COPD, but it differs from that seen in asthma [43,44]. Neutrophils, macrophages, and $CD8^+$ T lymphocytes are increased in the airways of patients who have COPD rather than the eosinophils and $CD4^+$ lymphocytes seen in asthma. Activated neutrophils and macrophages release proteases and reactive oxygen species, both of which have been implicated in the lung parenchymal destruction that defines emphysema. Increased neutrophils in the sputum of patients with COPD are associated with a more rapid decline in lung function [45]. In smokers, the number of inflammatory cells in airway tissue correlated inversely with FEV_1 (r = −0.7, $P = 0.005$) and directly with radiographic emphysema (r = 0.8, $P < 0.005$) [46]. It is logical that if PM exposure increases neutrophil influx into the airways of smokers or others susceptible to COPD, it may enhance the progression of, or risk for, the disease.

Few data are available on the inflammatory response to PM exposure in people who have COPD. Gong and colleagues [47] found small reductions in oxygen saturation but no increases in inflammatory cells in induced sputum after inhalation of concentrated ambient fine PM in subjects who have COPD. Similarly, no inflammatory effects were observed with exposures to concentrated coarse PM [48]. People who have COPD may be at increased risk from PM effects because of impaired functional status at baseline, however.

People who have COPD also have systemic inflammation. Tumor necrosis factor-α and its receptors, interleukin-6, and interleukin-8 are increased in the blood of patients who have COPD and increase further with exacerbations [49]. Smoking has similar effects. These mediators of the systemic inflammatory response, also known as the acute phase response, contribute in the pathogenesis of atherosclerotic vascular disease and place patients who have COPD at increased risk for cardiovascular events.

The obstructive lung diseases that place people at increased risk for mortality and morbidity from PM exposure—asthma and COPD—are inflammatory diseases. Severe exacerbations of asthma and COPD are treated with corticosteroids, which are potent anti-inflammatory agents. If PM exposures enhance airway inflammation in these diseases, it would be expected to worsen their course.

Smoking

Cigarette smoke contains particulate matter and gases produced by the combustion of tobacco and its additives. It contains more than 4000 individual chemical species, many of which are known to be harmful to the respiratory, cardiovascular, and other systems. Inflammation is integral to the adverse effects of either direct or indirect exposure to cigarette smoke, and smoking-related disease serves as a model for the health effects of exposure to PM in ambient air, either outdoors or in the workplace.

Chronic cigarette smoking causes increased neutrophilic inflammation in the airways. There is increased recovery of neutrophils in induced sputum and in bronchoalveolar lavage fluid from active smokers. There is evidence that reactive oxygen species and proteolytic enzymes released from activated neutrophils in the lung contribute to the pathogenesis of COPD. Exposure to PM and other pollutants may enhance this oxidant burden. For example, cigarette smoking increases the number of alveolar macrophages in the lung more than threefold, and these macrophages may have increased potential to release reactive oxygen species in response to pollutant exposure [50]. Permeability of the alveolar epithelium, as measured by the clearance rate of inhaled diethylenetriaminepentaacetate (DTPA), is increased in smokers and returns toward normal with smoking cessation [51,52]. This "leakiness" of the pulmonary alveolar epithelium is likely a consequence of toxins in smoke itself and the inflammation that accompanies the injury.

Whether the underlying airway inflammation in smokers confers an increased risk for health effects of long-term PM exposure is unclear. In the recent analysis of PM mortality effects using the American Cancer Society database [53], the absolute risks of air pollution for cardiovascular mortality were larger for smokers than for nonsmokers, which suggests that the cardiovascular risks of PM exposure were at least additive to the risks of smoking itself. This was not true for the association between PM exposure and respiratory causes of mortality, which was not increased in smokers relative to nonsmokers. Thus, PM exposure likely exacerbates underlying respiratory disease in smokers and nonsmokers but may increase the progression of various cardiovascular diseases, more so in smokers.

Inflammation and atherosclerosis

The effects of PM exposure in cardiovascular disease are addressed by Godleski elsewhere in this issue and are not discussed in detail here. It is important to recognize, however, that atherosclerosis, the underlying cause of most cardiovascular mortality, is an inflammatory disease.

The current paradigm in the pathogenesis of the atherosclerotic plaque assigns a key role to oxidants, circulating leukocytes, and low-density lipoprotein (LDL) [54]. LDL accumulates in the subendothelial space of the vessel and is partially oxidized by reactive oxygen species produced by local monocytes, polymorphonuclear leukocytes (PMN), and macrophages. Oxidized LDL inhibits NO synthesis by endothelial cells, apparently by intracellular translocation of endothelial nitric oxide synthase (NOS) [55]. It also increases adhesiveness of PMN [56], enhances reactive oxygen species production by leukocytes [57], and activates monocytes for production of monocyte chemotactic protein-1 and interleukin-8 [58]. This leads to further monocyte recruitment and further LDL oxidation. Oxidized LDL is recognized by the scavenger receptor of monocytes and is avidly ingested to form the "foam cells" characteristic of the maturing atherosclerotic plaque. Lymphocytes within the plaque demonstrate activation, with increased expression of CD25, an epitope of the interleukin-2 receptor.

Endothelial dysfunction is the underlying and earliest abnormality in atherosclerotic vascular disease [59]. A healthy endothelium maintains vascular homeostasis, including control of blood pressure, regulation of leukocyte traffic, and control of thrombosis [60], primarily through production of NO via action of NOS on L-arginine. Endothelial cells produce endothelial NOS but can be induced to express inducible NOS [61]. Local NO release by endothelial cells diffuses to vascular smooth muscle to maintain vasodilatation and diffuses into the blood, where it reduces platelet adhesion and aggregation, reduces leukocyte adhesiveness and expression of adhesion molecules, downregulates leukocyte NADPH oxidase function, scavenges superoxide anion (O_2^-) [62], and prevents coagulation by inhibiting tissue factor expression in endothelial cells. NO also reacts quickly with hemoglobin and plasma proteins. These complex interactions may allow NO to regulate vascular tone in response to hypoxia via release of nitrite [63]. Many of these effects are opposed by endothelin-1, a potent vasoconstrictor that increases monocyte adhesion, promotes retention of PMN in the lung, and activates macrophages [64,65].

Elegant physiologic studies have demonstrated that vasodilatation in response to physiologic stimuli (eg, shear stress) is mediated by NO and that abnormal endothelial function or responsiveness is essentially a functional NO deficiency state that allows vasoconstrictors such as endothelins to predominate. Endothelial NO is reduced in cigarette smoking, diabetes, hyperlipidemia, and atherosclerosis [59]. Endothelial function is abnormal in these states, and this dysfunction precedes the development of atherosclerotic plaques. Chronic inhibition of NO synthase exacerbates atherogenesis in animal models [66]. Administration of L-arginine (to increase NO production via NOS) was anti-atherogenic in rabbits [67], normalized leukocyte adhesion [68], improved endothelial function in patients with atherosclerosis

[54], improved coronary endothelial function in patients with nonobstructive coronary artery disease [69], and normalized the myocardial blood flow response to the cold pressor test in smokers [70].

Superoxide and other reactive species are released in the inflamed vascular wall by leukocytes and may be generated by reactive chemical species delivered on the surface of inhaled particles [71]. Depletion of NO occurs in part because of NO reactions with O_2^-, which produce peroxynitrite, a strong oxidant. O_2^- and peroxynitrite participate in the oxidation of LDL, with further damage to the endothelium. Administration of antioxidant vitamins improves endothelial function by scavenging reactive oxygen species and increasing functional NO levels.

One of the key unresolved questions regarding cardiovascular effects of PM exposure is whether the cardiovascular effects are a consequence of pulmonary inflammation. In human clinical studies, the absence of changes in pulmonary function, inflammatory cells in induced sputum, and increases in airway NO production argue against significant inflammatory effects of fine and ultrafine PM in the conducting airways. The single study that used bronchoalveolar lavage indicated that CAPs exposure induces inflammation in the distal airways or alveolar space [8]. This finding was supported by epidemiologic studies that showed associations between increases in ambient PM and exhaled NO concentrations [28]. The inflammatory effects of PM at concentrations comparable to those in ambient air seem to be relatively mild and may not explain the epidemiologic findings of increased cardiovascular mortality and morbidity associated with PM exposure. It is likely that other, more direct mechanisms also play a role.

Particle characteristics and inflammation

It is likely that specific particle characteristics influence particle toxicity and inflammatory potential. Among the important characteristics are mass, number, size, surface area, solubility, chemical composition, chemical availability, biologic content, and ability to generate reactive oxygen and nitrogen species. Many of these particle characteristics are interrelated. For example, UFPs generally have increased capacity to generate reactive oxygen species in comparison with larger, fine particles, and this phenomenon is likely related to the large surface area of ultrafines, which serves as a "sink" for reactive organic vapors. On the other hand, coarse particles may have a greater content of biologically active materials, such as lipopolysaccharide. Instillation of the coarse fraction of PM_{10} into rat lungs caused greater PMN influx than did the fine fraction [72]. In this study, the inflammatory potential of the particles correlated best with their lipopolysaccharide content and not with metals or reactive oxygen species.

Clarke and colleagues [73] examined responses in healthy dogs to 6-hour inhalations of CAPs in Boston. The dogs were exposed via tracheostomy, and inflammation was assessed by inflammatory cell recovery in bronchoalveolar lavage fluid and numbers of leukocytes in blood. There was no significant relationship between particle mass and any of the inflammatory parameters. When the day-to-day variability in concentrated particle chemical composition was taken into account using a rotating factor analysis, however, significant relationships were observed between particle composition and inflammatory markers. For example, the number of neutrophils in bronchoalveolar lavage fluid was associated with increases in the aluminum/silicon factor; the number of blood neutrophils was associated with the vanadium/nickel factor. Decreases in blood hemoglobin levels were correlated with the sulfur factor. These findings suggested that physiologic effects of PM exposure may shift with changes in particle source and chemical composition. It is not possible to ascribe specific health effects to any of the identified factors or chemical components in the complex mix of ambient particles, however.

There is evidence for a role of transition metal content in mediating local inflammation. Epidemiologic studies in the Utah Valley demonstrated reduced health impacts of air pollution during closure of a local steel mill [74]. A series of studies have examined the relative toxicity of the ambient air particles collected in the Utah Valley before, during, and after the closure of the mill. Particles collected during the closure showed reduced inflammatory potential in vitro [75,76] and in vivo [77,78] in comparison with particles collected during operation. The reduced inflammatory potential corresponded to a reduced content of metals in the particle extract. Similarly, particles collected in Hettstedt, Germany, an area with extensive industrial activity and an increased prevalence of asthma in children, were compared with particles in a nonindustrialized area (Zerbst) by instilling them into the airways of healthy volunteers [79]. Hettstedt but not Zerbst particles caused an increase in monocytes in the bronchoalveolar lavage fluid and increased the reactive oxygen species generation by stimulated bronchoalveolar lavage cells. As in the Utah Valley studies, the Hettstedt particles had a higher content of transition metals than the Zerbst particles. In some in vitro studies, toxicity was reduced with chelation of metals [80,81].

Other studies have suggested that reactive organic species may be important in inducing injury and inflammation. Organic fractions of DEP can activate inflammatory responses in airway epithelial cells [82] and have been shown to activate heme-oxygenase-1 and other redox-active enzymes in macrophages and epithelial cells [83,84]. Organic components of PM also have been implicated in cardiovascular effects. Hospital admissions for coronary artery disease were increased in areas contaminated with persistent organic pollutants [85]. Phenanthroquinone, an organic component of DEP, reduced expression of endothelial nitric oxide synthase, reduced vasodilatation of aortic rings, and elevated blood pressure when injected intraperitoneally in rats [86]. Environmental aldehydes may be cardiotoxic and increase the progression of atherosclerosis [87].

UFPs have an increased potential for the induction of inflammation when compared on an equal mass basis with larger particles [88].

Hypotheses to explain this occurrence have focused on the high surface area of UFPs, which may serve to carry organic molecules and reactive oxygen and nitrogen species into the deep lung. Elder and colleagues [89] examined the interaction of inhalation of elemental carbon particles with a known inflammatory stimulus—endotoxin—in elderly and hypertensive rats. Carbon UFPs alone did not cause airway inflammation but significantly modified the systemic inflammatory response to endotoxin, with enhancement of PMN production of reactive oxygen species. This finding indicated that even relatively inert carbon UFPs may enhance aspects of the inflammatory response to infectious agents.

Recent evidence shows that UFPs differ from larger particles in the way they enter cells: they seem to be able to diffuse through the lipid cell membrane and enter free into the cytoplasm, not enclosed in a membrane vesicle [90]. From there they can enter the nucleus or mitochondria and interfere with cellular energy processes. They can cross the epithelium, enter vascular endothelial cells and even red blood cells, and possibly be transported via the blood to other organs. The translocation of UFPs beyond the lung is discussed in more detail in this issue by Elder and Oberdörster.

The particle mix on roadways seems to induce inflammatory effects. Mild pulmonary inflammatory responses were seen in a study of "on-road" exposures to ambient particles in rats [91,92]. In one experiment, a single 6-hour exposure to on-road aerosols was found to increase the total number of cells in bronchoalveolar fluid 3 days after exposure in comparison to filtered air controls. In a separate experiment, the aerosols were found to induce a decrease in the percentage of circulating PMNs relative to filtered air controls after a single 6-hour exposure regardless of pretreatment (lipopolysaccharide or saline aerosol given immediately before on-road exposures). On-road aerosols also were found to decrease the concentration of plasma fibrinogen in rats exposed for 3 consecutive days and then euthanized 3 days after the last exposure.

The pulmonary inflammatory response to PM exposure may be related in part to organic components of PM and the generation of reactive oxygen species. The relationship between the organic chemical composition and the redox cycling potential of ambient PM was confirmed in a study in which UFPs were compared with coarse and fine particles collected in the Los Angeles basin [93]. Ambient UFPs were more active in generating reactive oxygen species than coarse and fine particles and were more effective in inducing oxidative stress in macrophages. The in vitro and cellular responses showed a strong correlation with the polycyclic aromatic hydrocarbon content of UFPs. These data show differential particle toxicity based on size, composition, and subcellular localization.

Summary

Inflammation is a complex pathophysiologic process that is required for survival of the organism. It is a key component of defense against invading micro-organisms and repair of tissue injury. Inflammation is under complex genetic control, and the manifestations are local and systemic. Inflammatory injury of host tissues and organs is tightly linked with the generation of reactive oxygen species and antioxidant defense (see article in this issue by Xia and colleagues). Underlying lung diseases that involve inflammation, such as asthma and COPD, may be worsened when inhalation of ambient PM enhances inflammatory responses. There is growing evidence that exposure to traffic emissions, especially diesel exhaust, may worsen asthma and enhance allergen responsiveness. Inflammation is also central to the development of atherosclerotic vascular disease, and PM exposure may accelerate that process. PM exposure may have acute effects on endothelial function in pulmonary and systemic vascular beds. Particle composition and physical characteristics are likely to determine PM inflammatory potential and toxicity. Key PM characteristics hypothesized to promote inflammatory responses are size and surface area, metal content, organic content, and ability to generate reactive oxygen species. Sorting out the important characteristics has only just begun, however.

References

[1] Kumar V, Abbas AK, Fausto N. Acute and chronic inflammation. In: Kumar V, Abbas AK, Fausto N, editors. Robbins and Cotran pathologic basis of disease. 7th edition. New York: Elsevier Saunders; 2005. p. 47–86.

[2] Torres A, Utell MJ, Morrow PE, et al. Airway inflammation in smokers and nonsmokers with varying responsiveness to ozone. Am J Respir Crit Care Med 1997;156:728–36.

[3] Peden DB. The epidemiology and genetics of asthma risk associated with air pollution. J Allergy Clin Immunol 2005;115(2):213–9.

[4] Gilliland FD, Li YF, Saxon A, et al. Effect of glutathione-S-transferase M1 and P1 genotypes on xenobiotic enhancement of allergic responses: randomised, placebo-controlled crossover study. Lancet 2004;363(9403):119–25.

[5] Beutler B. Science review: key inflammatory and stress pathways in critical illness. The central role of the Toll-like receptors. Crit Care 2003;7(1):39–46.

[6] Calvano SE, Xiao W, Richards DR, et al. A network-based analysis of systemic inflammation in humans. Nature 2005;437(7061):1032–7.

[7] Cobb JP, Mindrinos MN, Miller-Graziano C, et al. Application of genome-wide expression analysis to human health and disease. Proc Natl Acad Sci U S A 2005;102(13): 4801–6.

[8] Ghio AJ, Kim C, Devlin RB. Concentrated ambient air particles induce mild pulmonary inflammation in healthy human volunteers. Am J Respir Crit Care Med 2000; 162:981–8.

[9] Gong H Jr, Linn WS, Sioutas C, et al. Controlled exposures of healthy and asthmatic volunteers to concentrated ambient fine particles in Los Angeles. Inhal Toxicol 2003;15:305–25.

[10] Pietropaoli AP, Frampton MW, Hyde RW, et al. Pulmonary function, diffusing capacity and inflammation in healthy and asthmatic subjects exposed to ultrafine particles. Inhal Toxicol 2004;16(Suppl 1):59–72.

[11] Pietropaoli AP, Frampton MW, Oberdörster G, et al. Blood markers of coagulation and inflammation in healthy human subjects exposed to carbon ultrafine particles. In: Heinrich U, editor. Effects of air contaminants on the respiratory tract: interpretations from molecular to meta analysis. Stuttgart: Fraunhofer IRB Verlag; 2004. p. 181–94.

[12] Saldiva PHN, Clarke RW, Coull BA, et al. Lung inflammation induced by concentrated ambient air particles is related to particle composition. Am J Respir Crit Care Med 2002;165: 1610–7.

[13] Lippmann M, Gordon T, Chen LC. Effects of subchronic exposures to concentrated ambient particles in mice. IX. Integral assessment and human health implications of subchronic exposures of mice to CAPs. Inhal Toxicol 2005;17(4–5):255–61.

[14] Nowak D, Jorres R, Berger J, et al. Airway responsiveness to sulfur dioxide in an adult population sample. Am J Respir Crit Care Med 1997;156(4 Pt 1):1151–6.

[15] Platts-Mills TA. The role of immunoglobulin E in allergy and asthma. Am J Respir Crit Care Med 2001;164(8 Pt 2):S1–5.

[16] Platts-Mills TA. The role of allergens in the induction of asthma. Curr Allergy Asthma Rep 2002;2(2):175–80.

[17] Brown JS, Zeman KL, Bennett WD. Ultrafine particle deposition and clearance in the healthy and obstructed lung. Am J Respir Crit Care Med 2002;166:1240–7.

[18] Chalupa DC, Morrow PE, Oberdörster G, et al. Ultrafine particle deposition in subjects with asthma. Environ Health Perspect 2004;112:879–82.

[19] Peden DB, Boehlecke B, Horstman D, et al. Prolonged acute exposure to 0.16 ppm ozone induces eosinophilic airway inflammation in asthmatic subjects with allergies. J Allergy Clin Immunol 1997;100(6 Pt 1):802–8.

[20] Jörres R, Nowak D, Magnussen H. The effect of ozone exposure on allergen responsiveness in subjects with asthma or rhinitis. Am J Respir Crit Care Med 1996;153:56–64.

[21] Kehrl HR, Peden DB, Ball B, et al. Increased specific airway reactivity of persons with mild allergic asthma after 7.6 hours of exposure to 0.16 ppm ozone. J Allergy Clin Immunol 1999; 104(6):1198–204.

[22] Thurston GD, Lippmann M, Scott MB, et al. Summertime haze air pollution and children with asthma. Am J Respir Crit Care Med 1997;155:654–60.

[23] Pope CA, Dockery DW, Spengler JD, et al. Respiratory health and PM_{10} pollution. Am Rev Respir Dis 1991;144:668–74.

[24] Dusseldorp A, Kruize H, Brunekreef B, et al. Associations of PM10 and airborne iron with respiratory health of adults living near a steel factory. Am J Respir Crit Care Med 1995;152: 1932–9.

[25] Utell MJ, Morrow PE, Speers DM, et al. Airway responses to sulfate and sulfuric acid aerosols in asthmatics: an exposure-response relationship. Am Rev Respir Dis 1983;128: 444–50.

[26] Frampton MW, Morrow PE, Cox C, et al. Sulfuric acid aerosol followed by ozone exposure in healthy and asthmatic subjects. Environ Res 1995;69:1–14.

[27] Linn WS, Anderson KR, Shamoo DA, et al. Controlled exposures of young asthmatics to mixed oxidant gases and acid aerosol. Am J Respir Crit Care Med 1995;152:885–91.

[28] Koenig JQ, Jansen K, Mar TF, et al. Measurement of offline exhaled nitric oxide in a study of community exposure to air pollution. Environ Health Perspect 2003;111(13):1625–9.

[29] Pandya RJ, Solomon G, Kinner A, et al. Diesel exhaust and asthma: hypotheses and molecular mechanisms of action. Environ Health Perspect 2002;110:103–12.

[30] Koren HS, Utell MJ. Asthma and the environment. Environ Health Perspect 1997;105: 534–7.

[31] Brauer M, Hoek G, Van Vliet P, et al. Air pollution from traffic and the development of respiratory infections and asthmatic and allergic symptoms in children. Am J Respir Crit Care Med 2002;166(8):1092–8.

[32] Janssen NAH, Brunekreef B, van Vliet P, et al. The relationship between air pollution from heavy traffic and allergic sensitization, bronchial hyperresponsiveness, and respiratory symptoms in Dutch schoolchildren. Environ Health Perspect 2003;111:1512–8.

[33] Edwards J, Walters S, Griffiths RK. Hospital admissions for asthma in pre-school children: relationship to major roads in Birmingham, United Kingdom. Arch Environ Health 1994;49: 223–7.

[34] Oosterlee A, Drijver M, Lebret E, et al. Chronic respiratory symptoms in children and adults living along streets with high traffic density. Occup Environ Med 1996;53(4):241–7.

[35] van Vliet P, Knape M, de Hartog J, et al. Motor vehicle exhaust and chronic respiratory symptoms in children living near freeways. Environ Res 1997;74(2):122–32.

[36] Salvi S, Blomberg A, Rudell B, et al. Acute inflammatory responses in the airways and peripheral blood after short-term exposure to diesel exhaust in healthy human volunteers. Am J Respir Crit Care Med 1999;159(3):702–9.

[37] Salvi SS, Nordenhall C, Blomberg A, et al. Acute exposure to diesel exhaust increases IL-8 and GRO-α production in healthy human airways. Am J Respir Crit Care Med 2000;161: 550–7.

[38] Nordenhäll C, Pourazar J, Ledin MC, et al. Diesel exhaust enhances airway responsiveness in asthmatic subjects. Eur Respir J 2001;17:909–15.

[39] Diaz-Sanchez D, Dotson AR, Takenaka H, et al. Diesel exhaust particles induce local IgE production in vivo and alter the pattern of IgE messenger RNA isoforms. J Clin Invest 1994;94:1417–25.

[40] Diaz-Sanchez D, Tsien A, Casillas A, et al. Enhanced nasal cytokine production in human beings after in vivo challenge with diesel exhaust particles. J Allergy Clin Immunol 1996;98: 114–23.

[41] Diaz-Sanchez D, Tsien A, Fleming J, et al. Combined diesel exhaust particulate and ragweed allergen challenge markedly enhances human in vivo nasal ragweed-specific IgE and skews cytokine production to a T helper cell 2-type pattern. J Immunol 1997;158:2406–13.

[42] Weinberger SE. Medical progress: recent advances in pulmonary medicine. N Engl J Med 1993;328:1389–97.

[43] Sutherland ER, Martin RJ. Airway inflammation in chronic obstructive pulmonary disease: comparisons with asthma. J Allergy Clin Immunol 2003;112(5):819–27 [quiz: 828].

[44] Wouters EF. Local and systemic inflammation in chronic obstructive pulmonary disease. Proc Am Thorac Soc 2005;2(1):26–33.

[45] Stanescu D, Sanna A, Veriter C, et al. Airways obstruction, chronic expectoration, and rapid decline of FEV_1 in smokers are associated with increased levels of sputum neutrophils. Thorax 1996;51:267–71.

[46] Turato G, Zuin R, Miniati M, et al. Airway inflammation in severe chronic obstructive pulmonary disease: relationship with lung function and radiologic emphysema. Am J Respir Crit Care Med 2002;166(1):105–10.

[47] Gong H Jr, Linn WS, Clark KW, et al. Respiratory responses to exposures with fine particulates and nitrogen dioxide in the elderly with and without COPD. Inhal Toxicol 2005;17(3): 123–32.

[48] Gong H Jr, Linn WS, Terrell SL, et al. Altered heart-rate variability in asthmatic and healthy volunteers exposed to concentrated ambient coarse particles. Inhal Toxicol 2004;16:335–43.

[49] van Eeden SF, Yeung A, Quinlam K, et al. Systemic response to ambient particulate matter: relevance to chronic obstructive pulmonary disease. Proc Am Thorac Soc 2005;2(1):61–7.

[50] Voter KZ, Whitin JC, Torres A, et al. Ozone exposure and the production of reactive oxygen species by bronchoalveolar cells in humans. Inhal Toxicol 2001;13:465–83.

[51] Minty BD, Jordan C, Jones JG. Rapid improvement in abnormal pulmonary epithelial permeability after stopping cigarettes. BMJ 1981;282:1183–6.

[52] Stewart JC, Hyde RW, Boscia J, et al. Changes in markers of epithelial permeability and inflammation in chronic smokers switching to a non-burning tobacco device (Eclipse). Nicotine Tob Res 2006, in press.

[53] Pope CAI, Burnett RT, Thurston GD, et al. Cardiovascular mortality and long-term exposure to particulate air pollution: epidemiological evidence of general pathophysiological pathways of disease. Circulation 2004;109:71–7.

[54] Diaz MN, Frei B, Vita JA, et al. Antioxidants and atherosclerotic heart disease. N Engl J Med 1997;337:408–16.

[55] Nuszkowski A, Grabner R, Marsche G, et al. Hypochlorite-modified low density lipoprotein inhibits nitric oxide synthesis in endothelial cells via an intracellular dislocalization of endothelial nitric-oxide synthase. J Biol Chem 2001;276(17):14212–21.

[56] Hazell LJ, Stocker R. Oxidation of low-density lipoprotein with hypochlorite causes transformation of the lipoprotein into a high-uptake form for macrophages. Biochem J 1993; 290(Pt 1):165–72.

[57] Kopprasch S, Leonhardt W, Pietzsch J, et al. Hypochlorite-modified low-density lipoprotein stimulates human polymorphonuclear leukocytes for enhanced production of reactive oxygen metabolites, enzyme secretion, and adhesion to endothelial cells. Atherosclerosis 1998; 136(2):315–24.

[58] Woenckhaus C, Kaufmann A, Bussfeld D, et al. Hypochlorite-modified LDL: chemotactic potential and chemokine induction in human monocytes. Clin Immunol Immunopathol 1998;86(1):27–33.

[59] Quyyumi AA. Endothelial function in health and disease: new insights into the genesis of cardiovascular disease. Am J Med 1998;105(1A):32S–9S.

[60] Pearson JD. Normal endothelial cell function. Lupus 2000;9(3):183–8.

[61] Cines DB, Pollak ES, Buck CA, et al. Endothelial cells in physiology and in the pathophysiology of vascular disorders. Blood 1998;91:3527–61.

[62] Lefer AM. Nitric oxide: nature's naturally occurring leukocyte inhibitor. Circulation 1997; 95(3):553–4.

[63] Gladwin MT, Schechter AN, Kim-Shapiro DB, et al. The emerging biology of the nitrite anion. Nat Chem Biol 2005;1:308–14.

[64] Mathew V, Hasdai D, Lerman A. The role of endothelin in coronary atherosclerosis. Mayo Clin Proc 1996;71:769–77.

[65] Sato Y, Hogg JC, English D, et al. Endothelin-1 changes polymorphonuclear leukocytes' deformability and CD11b expression and promotes their retention in the lung. Am J Respir Cell Mol Biol 2000;23:404–10.

[66] Maxwell AJ, Tsao PS, Cooke JP. Modulation of the nitric oxide synthase pathway in atherosclerosis. Exp Physiol 1998;83(5):573–84.

[67] Goumas G, Tentolouris C, Tousoulis D, et al. Therapeutic modification of the L-arginine-eNOS pathway in cardiovascular diseases. Atherosclerosis 2001;154(2):255–67.

[68] Brandes RP, Brandes S, Boger RH, et al. L-arginine supplementation in hypercholesterolemic rabbits normalizes leukocyte adhesion to non-endothelial matrix. Life Sci 2000; 66(16):1519–24.

[69] Lerman A, Burnett JC Jr, Higano ST, et al. Long-term L-arginine supplementation improves small-vessel coronary endothelial function in humans. Circulation 1998;97(21):2123–8.

[70] Campisi R, Czernin J, Schoder H, et al. L-Arginine normalizes coronary vasomotion in long-term smokers. Circulation 1999;99(4):491–7.

[71] Dick CA, Brown DM, Donaldson K, et al. The role of free radicals in the toxic and inflammatory effects of four different ultrafine particle types. Inhal Toxicol 2003;15(1):39–52.

[72] Schins RPF, Lightbody JH, Borm PJA, et al. Inflammatory effects of coarse and fine particulate matter in relation to chemical and biological constituents. Toxicol Appl Pharmacol 2004;195:1–11.

[73] Clarke RW, Coull B, Reinisch U, et al. Inhaled concentrated ambient particles are associated with hematologic and bronchoalveolar lavage changes in canines. Environ Health Perspect 2000;108:1179–87.

[74] Pope CA, Schwartz J, Ransom MR. Daily mortality and PM_{10} pollution in Utah Valley. Arch Environ Health 1992;47:211–7.

[75] Devlin RB, Ghio AJ, Samet JM, et al. Pulmonary toxicity of Utah Valley PM: are empirical indices of adverse health effects coherent with the epidemiology? In: Bates DV, Brain JD, Driscoll KE, et al, editors. Relationships between acute and chronic effects of air pollution. Washington, DC: ILSI Press; 2000. p. 159–68.

[76] Frampton MW, Ghio AJ, Samet JM, et al. Effects of aqueous extracts of PM_{10} filters from the Utah Valley on human airway epithelial cells. Am J Physiol 1999;277:L960–7.

[77] Dye JA, Lehmann JR, McGee JK, et al. Acute pulmonary toxicity of particulate matter filter extracts in rats: coherence with epidemiologic studies in Utah Valley residents. Environ Health Perspect 2001;109(Suppl 3):395–403.

[78] Ghio AJ, Devlin RB. Inflammatory lung injury after bronchial instillation of air pollution particles. Am J Respir Crit Care Med 2001;164:704–8.

[79] Schaumann F, Borm PJA, Herbrich A, et al. Metal-rich ambient particles (particulate matter$_{2.5}$) cause airway inflammation in healthy subjects. Am J Respir Crit Care Med 2004;170: 898–903.

[80] Prahalad AK, Inmon J, Dailey LA, et al. Air pollution particles mediated oxidative DNA base damage in a cell free system and in human airway epithelial cells in relation to particulate metal content and bioreactivity. Chem Res Toxicol 2001;14(7):879–87.

[81] Knaapen AM, Shi T, Borm PJ, et al. Soluble metals as well as the insoluble particle fraction are involved in cellular DNA damage induced by particulate matter. Mol Cell Biochem 2002; 234–235(1–2):317–26.

[82] Bonvallot V, Baeza-Squiban A, Baulig A, et al. Organic compounds from diesel exhaust particles elicit a proinflammatory response in human airway epithelial cells and induce cytochrome p450 1A1 expression. Am J Respir Cell Mol Biol 2001;25:515–21.

[83] Li N, Venkatesan MI, Miguel A, et al. Induction of heme oxygenase-1 expression in macrophages by diesel exhaust particle chemicals and quinones via the antioxidant-responsive element. J Immunol 2000;165:3393–401.

[84] Li N, Alam J, Venkatesan MI, et al. Nrf2 is a key transcription factor that regulates antioxidant defense in macrophages and epithelial cells: protecting against the proinflammatory and oxidizing effects of diesel exhaust chemicals. J Immunol 2004;173(5):3467–81.

[85] Sergeev AV, Carpenter DO. Hospitalization rates for coronary heart disease in relation to residence near areas contaminated with persistent organic pollutants and other pollutants. Environ Health Perspect 2005;113:756–61.

[86] Kumagai Y, Hayashi T, Miyauchi T, et al. Phenanthroquinone inhibits eNOS activity and suppresses vasorelaxation. Am J Physiol 2001;281:R25–30.

[87] Bhatnagar A. Cardiovascular pathophysiology of environmental pollutants. Am J Physiol Heart Circ Physiol 2004;286(2):H479–85.

[88] Oberdörster G. Pulmonary effects of inhaled ultrafine particles. Int Arch Occup Environ Health 2001;74:1–8.

[89] Elder ACP, Gelein R, Azadniv M, et al. Systemic effects of inhaled ultrafine particles in two compromised, aged rat strains. Inhal Toxicol 2004;16:461–71.

[90] Geiser M, Rothen-Rutishauser B, Kapp N, et al. Ultrafine particles cross cellular membranes by nonphagocytic mechanisms in lungs and in cultured cells. Environ Health Perspect 2005; 113(11):1555–60.

[91] Elder A, Gelein R, Finkelstein J, et al. On-road exposure to highway aerosols. 2. Exposures of aged, compromised rats. Inhal Toxicol 2004;16(Suppl 1):41–53.

[92] Kittelson DB, Watts WF, Johnson JP, et al. On-road exposure to highway aerosols. 1. Aerosol and gas measurements. Inhal Toxicol 2004;16(Suppl 1):31–9.

[93] Li N, Sioutas C, Cho A, et al. Ultrafine particulate pollutants induce oxidative stress and mitochondrial damage. Environ Health Perspect 2003;111:455–60.

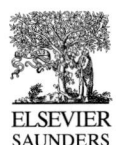

ELSEVIER
SAUNDERS

Clin Occup Environ Med
5 (4) 817–836

CLINICS IN
OCCUPATIONAL AND
ENVIRONMENTAL
MEDICINE

The Role of Reactive Oxygen Species and Oxidative Stress in Mediating Particulate Matter Injury

Tian Xia, MD, PhD[a,b], Michael Kovochich, BS[a,b], Andre Nel, MD, PhD[a,b,*]

[a]Division of Clinical Immunology and Allergy, Department of Medicine,
University of California Los Angeles, 52-175 CHS, 10833 Le Conte Avenue,
Los Angeles, CA 90095-1680, USA
[b]Southern California Particle Center, 650 Charles E. Young Drive South,
Box 951772, Los Angeles, CA 90095-1772, USA

Several plausible mechanisms have been proposed to explain the adverse health effects of particulate matter (PM) in polluted ambient air [1]. To date, experimental support has been provided for the role of local and systemic inflammation, cytokine and chemokine production, increased bone marrow production of myeloid lineage cells, free oxygen radical production in the chest, endotoxin-mediated cellular and tissue responses, stimulation of irritant receptors, and covalent modification of key cellular enzymes [1,2]. Best characterized in humans are the effects of PM on airway inflammation [3]. Several human and animal studies have shown that inhalation of diesel exhaust particles (DEP), a model particulate pollutant, and concentrated ambient particles elicit proinflammatory effects, cytokine production, and enhancement of allergic responses in the upper and lower airways [2–4]. The mechanistic link between the PM exposure and inflammation depends

Support for this article provided by US Public Health Service grants U19AI 070453 (UCLA Asthma and Allergic Disease Clinical Research Center), RO1 ES10553 (National Institute of Environmental and Health Science), RO1 ES15498, RO1 ES13432, and RO1 ES10253 and the US Environmental Protection Agency STAR award (RD-83241301) to the Southern California Particle Center and Supersite. This work has not been subjected to the Environmental Protection Agency for peer and policy review and does not necessarily reflect the views of the agency. No official endorsement should be inferred.

* Corresponding author. Division of Clinical Immunology and Allergy, Department of Medicine, University of California Los Angeles, 52-175 CHS, 10833 Le Conte Avenue, Los Angeles, CA 90095-1680.

E-mail address: anel@mednet.ucla.edu (A. Nel).

doi:10.1016/j.coem.2006.07.005

on generation of reactive oxygen species (ROS) and oxidative stress [2,5–7]. Although there is still debate about which particle components are responsible for ROS generation, there is accumulating evidence that pro-oxidative organic chemical compounds and transition metals play a role in ROS production [8,9]. The large reactive surface area of ambient ultrafine particles (UFP) also may play a role in ROS generation [10]. Target cells such as airway epithelial cells and macrophages also generate ROS in response to particle components by involving biologic processes [2,6,8].

ROS are capable of damaging key cellular components. To defend against this damage, cells use glutathione (GSH) and other high molecular weight antioxidants to inactivate oxygen radicals and protect cellular components against damage. In the setting of overwhelming ROS production, GSH depletion can induce a state of redox stress (ie, oxidative stress in the cell) [2,11]. Oxidative stress acts as a trigger that initiates a series of cellular responses, which can either be protective (eg, induction of antioxidant enzymes) or injurious in nature [12]. In this article we discuss the mechanisms and particle characteristics that contribute to ROS production and oxidative stress, including the experimental and clinical evidence that oxidative stress leads to clinically relevant disease. Finally, we review the biology of oxidative stress to explain the pathogenesis of PM-induced adverse health effects.

Evidence that reactive oxygen species and oxidative stress are involved in particular matter–induced injury

The principal target organs for PM-induced injury are the lung and the cardiovascular system. Pulmonary effects include small airway inflammation, which can lead to the exacerbation of asthma and chronic bronchitis, airway obstruction, and decreased gas exchange [2,13,14]. PM also can interfere with the clearance and inactivation of bacteria in the lung, which can lead to respiratory tract infection. There is growing awareness that PM is also a cardiovascular risk factor that is involved in heart attacks, stroke, rhythm disturbances, and sudden death [15]. Emerging evidence suggests that that some of these cardiovascular effects can be explained by enhanced atherogenesis and by systemic proinflammatory effects that impact the endothelium and blood coagulation pathways [15]. A common injury mechanism that links cardiovascular and pulmonary adverse health effects is PM-induced inflammation. We discuss the possibility that these proinflammatory effects constitute an oxidative stress response that is related to the ability of PM to induce ROS generation in specific airway and vascular target tissue.

In vitro evidence for the ability of PM to induce oxidative stress has emerged from several studies using DEP as a model air pollutant. Exposure of macrophages and bronchial epithelial cells, two of the principal targets for PM in the lung, to DEP leads to increased H_2O_2 and superoxide ($O_2^\bullet$) production in a time- and dose-dependant manner [16–18]. The kinetics of ROS generation in macrophages exhibit two phases, namely an early phase of mostly H_2O_2 production, followed by a later phase of $O_2^{\bullet-}$ production [16,17]. These phases could reflect different biologic events, as is discussed later. Intact particles and their methanol extracts can induce ROS production, which is accompanied by GSH depletion and induction of oxidative stress [17–19]. N-acetylcysteine (NAC), a thiol antioxidant, interferes in these cellular responses [7,20], further substantiating the role of oxidative stress in PM injury. Studies involving ambient concentrated particles, including ambient UFP, show similar effects on ROS production, GSH depletion, and induction of oxidative stress responses [8,21,22].

In vivo evidence for the ability of PM to induce ROS production and oxidative stress has been provided by using chemiluminescence sensors [21,22]. Using photomultiplier techniques, researchers demonstrated that H_2O_2 production increases in a time- and dose-dependent manner over the mediastinum of rats receiving concentrated ambient particles [21,22]. This effect was accompanied by decreased heart rate variability and the generation of thiobarbituric reactive substances in that organ [21,22]. These effects were inhibited by NAC, which further suggested the importance of oxidative stress after PM exposure [21,22]. Another approach involves using electron spin resonance to detect ROS generation on particles and in biologic tissue that come into contact with particles [19,23]. This approach includes the detection of oxygen radicals by spin trap markers in the bronchoalveolar lavage fluid of rats receiving intratracheal DEP [24]. Indirect evidence for the role of oxidative stress in vivo comes from studies that examine the adjuvant effects of DEP in a murine model of allergic inflammation and asthma [20]. These adjuvant effects include increased ovalbumin-specific IgE production in mice exposed to DEP plus ovalbumin [20]. The thiol antioxidants, NAC and bucillamine, were found to be effective inhibitors of these pro-oxidative and adjuvant effects of DEP [20]. Research also has shown that treatment of mice with DEP increased nitric oxide (NO) production and NO synthase (iNOS) expression [6,25]. NO can combine with $O_2^{\bullet-}$ to generate the peroxynitrite ($ONOO^-$) radical, which can further damage the airway epithelium [26]. Pretreatment with N-G-monomethyl L-arginine, an iNOS inhibitor, significantly reduced the airway hyperresponsiveness induced by DEP [6].

There is limited evidence for the production of oxygen radicals and oxidative stress after PM exposure in humans. One study showed increased CO levels in the exhaled air of human subjects after exposure to DEP, likely reflecting the induction of heme oxygenase (HO-1) expression as a sensitive oxidative stress response protein [27]. HO-1 is an enzyme that is responsible for the catabolism of heme, leading to the generation of CO and biliverdin as catalytic products of that reaction [28]. NO in the expired air also has been shown to be a sensitive marker for assessment of inflammatory lung diseases [29]. Several human studies have shown that various components of air pollution are associated with increased levels of NO in exhaled air [30,31].

Particle components, including absorbed particulate matter chemicals, are responsible for spontaneous particulate matter–induced reactive oxygen species production

The mechanisms by which ambient PM generates ROS include biologic events and particle-induced redox chemistry. These events are key to understanding disease pathogenesis and PM toxicity. Although there has been much debate about whether the particles or their absorbed chemicals are responsible for PM injury, it is our view that the particles and their absorbed chemicals play important roles in ROS production. This notion is derived from the observations that PM (1) contains organic and inorganic chemical compounds that are capable of ROS generation [8,32], (2) can spontaneously generate $O_2^{\bullet-}$ and hydroxyl radicals ($^{\bullet}OH$) in the absence of a biologic catalyst [8,33], and (3) size and reactive surface area are independent physical variables that influence PM ability to generate oxidative stress and inflammation in experimental animals (Table 1) [8,10].

Emerging evidence indicates that particle size, surface area, and chemical composition are the chief characteristics that determine PM health risks [12]. Based on size, PM can be classified into coarse, fine, or ultrafine particles (Table 1) [10]. Coarse particles, which have an aerodynamic diameter of 2.5 to 10 μm, are mostly derived from soil and sea salts. Fine particles, which range in diameter from 0.1 to 2.5 μm, and UFP, with diameters <0.1 μm, are predominantly derived from fossil fuel combustion processes. Combustion particles are comprised of a carbonaceous core that consists of elemental carbon, which is coated with a layer of chemicals, including organic hydrocarbons, metals, nitrates, and sulfates [11,34]. Although several chemical components could contribute to particle toxicity, the principal components that are responsible for ROS production are transition metals and redox cycling organic chemical compounds [12,18,35].

Table 1
Characterization of different sized particles

	Coarse (PM$_{10}$)	Fine (PM$_{2.5}$)	Ultrafine
Particle size	2.5–10 μm	0.1–2.5 μm	<100 nm
Particle number/mass	+	++	+++
Surface area	+	++	+++
Carbon content (elemental)	+	++	+++
Carbon content (organic)	+	++	+++
Metals	+++	++	+
PAH content	+	++	+++
Redox activity (DTT assay)	+	++	+++

Abbreviations: DTT, dithiothreitol; PAH, polycyclic aromatic hydrocarbons.
Data from Li N, Sioutas C, Cho A, et al. Ultrafine particulate pollutants induce oxidative stress and mitochondrial damage. Environ Health Perspect 2003;111(4):455–60; Donaldson K, Tran CL. Inflammation caused by particles and fibers. Inhal Toxicol 2002;14(1):5–27.

Transition metals, such as iron, copper, vanadium, chromium, nickel, and cobalt are responsible for the conversion of H_2O_2 into $^\bullet OH$ by the Fenton reaction:

$$Fe^{2+} + H_2O_2 \rightarrow Fe^{3+} + ^\bullet OH + OH^-$$

Catalytically active metals present on PM have been associated with oxidative stress in vitro and in vivo [36,37]. Residual oil fly ash contains high concentrations of transition metals and is often used as a model for the induction of ROS production and inflammation by transition metals. For instance, it has been shown that residual oil fly ash can activate mitogen-activated protein kinases and induce the expression of interleukin-8, interleukin-6, and tumor necrosis factor-α by a chelator-sensitive pathway [35]. The induction of inflammation in the rat lung and proinflammatory cytokines in human bronchial epithelial cells by ambient PM also can be reduced by treatment with metal chelators [36]. It is also interesting that the metal content of ambient PM varies according to particle size and source and may affect its ability to induce oxidative stress [8].

The discovery of the role of organic PM chemicals in ROS production is an outgrowth of the observation that methanol extracts made from DEP are capable of mimicking the pro-oxidative and proinflammatory effects of intact particles [18,38]. Chemical fractionation of organic DEP extracts by silica gel chromatography, using the elution principle of increasing polar solvents, has defined two major chemical groups that contribute to ROS production and oxidative stress [38,39]. The first is aromatic compounds, including polycyclic aromatic hydrocarbons (PAHs). PAHs are cyclical compounds that contain two to seven phenyl rings (Fig. 1). In the presence of cellular targets, such as bronchial epithelial cells, PAHs are capable of inducing oxidative stress after biotransformation by cytochrome P450 1A1, expoxide hydrolase, or dihydrodiol dehydrogenase [40]. These enzymes convert PAHs to redox cycling quinones (see later discussion). Organic DEP extracts have been shown to induce the expression of cytochrome P450 1A1 in bronchial epithelial cells and rat lungs [41]. The specific PAH profile of ambient PM varies with combustion source (eg, heavy duty and light duty diesel engines preferentially emit low and high molecular weight PAHs, respectively) [42]. This profile is of environmental importance because PAHs are semivolatile substances that can be released and repartition to the particle surfaces, depending on the ring size and environmental temperature [43]. Ambient UFPs, which to a large extent are derived from diesel exhaust emissions, exhibit a higher PAH content in the winter versus the summer months, which correlates with the increased propensity of ambient PM collected in winter months to generate oxidative stress [43]. Among the ambient particles collected in the Los Angeles basin, UFPs have a higher PAH content than coarse and fine particles, which could explain why UFPs have an increased propensity to generate oxidative stress in epithelial cells and macrophages [8]. Molecular

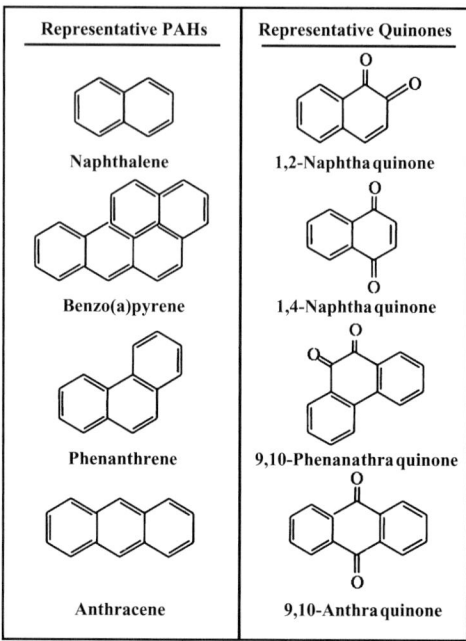

Fig. 1. Representative pro-oxidative organic chemical compounds, PAHs, and quinones. (*Modified from* Li N, Hao M, Phalen RF, et al. Particulate air pollutants and asthma: a paradigm for the role of oxidative stress in PM-induced adverse health effects. Clin Immunol 2003;109(3):254; with permission.)

epidemiologic studies in environmentally exposed populations also have shown that PAHs are linked to oxidative DNA damage, chromosome aberrations, formation of DNA adducts, and intrauterine growth retardation [44–46].

The second major class of organic chemical compounds that could contribute to PM-induced ROS production is polar substances, including oxidized forms of PAH (eg, ketones and quinones) [11,38]. The biologic mechanism by which quinones contribute to ROS generation is described in the section on biologic mechanisms.

In addition to providing a backbone for the adsorption of chemicals, the particle surface area and size are independent variables that determine ROS production and excitation of airway inflammation [47,48]. The same particle characteristics are also important in determining the pro-oxidative and proinflammatory effects of mineral dust particles and the generation of airway inflammation by experimental metal oxide particles [47,48]. There are several possible ways to explain these findings, including the fact that particle size is intimately linked to surface area. Table 2 shows the physical characteristics of a cloud of airborne particles of varying size but with a fixed mass of 10 $\mu g/m^3$ [10]. These calculations show that as the particle size

Table 2
Particle number and surface area varies with particle size as demonstrated for airborne particles with a fixed mass concentration of 10 $\mu g/m^3$

Particle diameter (μm)	Particles/cc in the air	Particle surface area ($\mu m^2/cc$)
2	1.2	24
0.5	153	120
0.02	2,400,000	3016

Data from Donaldson K, Tran CL. Inflammation caused by particles and fibers. Inhal Toxicol 2002;14(1):5–27.

decreases, the number of particles per unit air volume (1 cc) increases in exponential fashion, along with an exponential increase in the surface area. The increase in surface area places a larger number of potentially reactive chemical groups on the particle surface. This finding is of particular relevance to particles in the nano-size range (ie, UFPs), because the number of surface molecules is inversely related to the particle size. For instance, in a particle of 30-nm size, approximately 10% of the molecules are expressed on the surface, whereas at 10 and 3 nm, the ratios increase to 20% and 50%, respectively. The number of atoms or molecules on the particle surface determines characteristics such as electron storage and transfer to molecular dioxygen (O_2). At this stage it is unknown which chemicals or molecules are responsible for the formation of particle-associated reactive surface groups. What is known, however, is that even after organic extraction, the particulate core is still able to generate ROS, although in decreased amounts [49]. One possibility is that transition metals cooperate with electrophilic organic chemicals, such as quinone, to generate ROS on the particle surface [50], as demonstrated in Fig. 2.

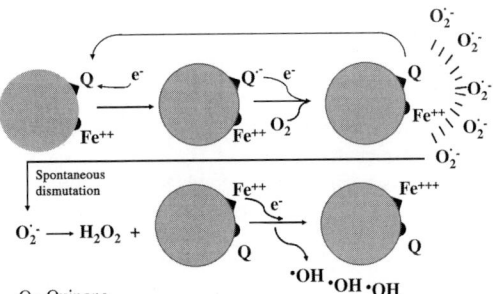

Fig. 2. Hypothetical model for particle-induced ROS production wherein organic chemicals cooperate with transition metals in the generation of the $^\bullet OH$ radical. Quinones can redox cycle on the particle surface. This reaction involves electron capture by the quinone (Q) to form a semiquinone. The semiquinone, in turn, transfer the electrons to O_2 molecule to generate $O_2^{\bullet-}$. Spontaneous dismutation of $O_2^{\bullet-}$ can lead to H_2O_2 production, which in the presence of ferrous ion on the particle surface can generate $^\bullet OH$ through the Fenton reaction.

Biologic mechanisms of particulate matter–induced reactive oxygen species generation

The origins of PM-induced ROS in biologic systems and target cells are from mixed subcellular sources (Fig. 3), including (1) catalytic conversion of PAHs to quinones by cytochrome P450 1A1 in the endoplasmic reticulum (Fig. 4), (2) quinone redox cycling by NADPH-dependent P450 reductase in microsomes (Fig. 4) [19], (3) mitochondrial perturbation leading to electron leakage in the inner membrane, and (4) NADPH oxidase activation on the cell membrane or the phagosome of macrophages.

Redox cycling organic chemicals are a major source of ROS generation in target tissue, such as bronchial epithelial cells, macrophages, and endothelial cells [17,51]. Quinones can act as catalysts to produce ROS during cellular responses to DEP [19]. Quinones are byproducts of diesel combustion and the enzymatic conversion of PAH in lung tissue [19]. Redox cycling

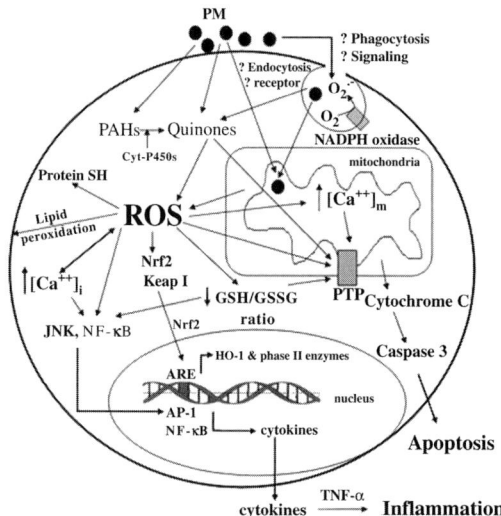

Fig. 3. Sources of ROS production and their effects on cells. Quinones can redox cycle to produce ROS in the endoplasmic reticulum under the catalytic influence of NADPH-cytochrome P450 reductase. Phagocytosis can induce the assembly and activation of NADPH oxidase to produce superoxide. PM can interfere in electron transduction in the mitochondrial inner membrane and in the perturbation of the PT pore to generate ROS. ROS leads to lipid peroxidation in the cell membrane and can crosslink protein SH groups and induce redox equilibrium through a depletion of GSH. Depending on the level of oxidative stress this could induce Nrf2 release to the nucleus, activation of mitogen-activated protein kinases and NF-κB signaling cascades, or cytotoxicity. Nrf2 interaction with the antioxidant response element leads to the expression of HO-1 and other phase II enzymes at low level of oxidative stress, whereas mitogen-activated protein kinases and NF-κB signaling cascades lead to proinflammatory responses (eg, cytokine production) at higher levels of oxidative stress. At the highest oxidative stress level, ROS can lead to opening of mitochondrial PT pore, followed by cytochrome c release, caspase-3 activation, and apoptosis or necrosis.

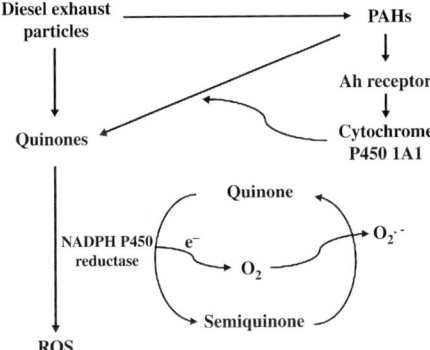

Fig. 4. PAHs can be converted to quinones by cytochrome P450 1A1. Reduction of quinones by NADPH P450 reductase leads to the formation of semiquinones, which are metastable and donate their electron to O_2 to form O_2^-. In the process, the original quinone is regenerated and can participate in several additional rounds of redox cycling. (*Modified from* Li N, Hao M, Phalen RF, et al. Particulate air pollutants and asthma: a paradigm for the role of oxidative stress in PM-induced adverse health effects. Clin Immunol 2003;109(3):254; with permission.)

quinones undergo one-electron reductions by NADPH cytochrome P450 reductase to form semiquinones (Fig. 4). The semiquinones are metastable and donate electrons to O_2, leading to the formation of $O_2^{\bullet-}$ as a byproduct [19]. In the process, the original quinones are being regenerated and can contribute to multiple rounds of $O_2^{\bullet-}$ generation (ie, redox cycle). Because of their high content of organic chemicals, ambient UFPs contribute proportionally more redox cycling chemicals than larger particles, as demonstrated by the increased ability of UFPs to generate $O_2^{\bullet-}$ in the dithiothreitol assay [8,33]. The dithiothreitol assay has been developed to measure the content of redox cycling chemicals present in fresh ambient PM samples collected by particle concentrators from ambient air [8,33].

Mitochondria are the main subcellular source of ROS production, even under physiologic conditions [52–54]. Mitochondria catalyze ATP production, which is linked to the activity of an electron transduction chain that operates in the inner membrane. This respiratory chain, which derives its electrons from NADH and $FADH_2$, consists of three multiprotein complexes in the inner membrane: the NADH dehydrogenase complex (I), the cytochrome c reductase complex (III), and the cytochrome c oxidase complex (IV). The chain also includes two diffusible molecules, ubiquinone and cytochrome c, which function as electron transporters between complexes I and III and between complexes III and IV, respectively. Electrons are transferred in a stepwise fashion along this chain, moving from a high to a low redox potential, which ultimately leads to the formation of H_2O [52–54]. The dissipation in electron energy during this "downhill" flow is used by the respiratory complexes (I, III, and IV) to pump protons (H^+) from the matrix into the intermembrane space against a concentration gradient. This event leads to the formation of the mitochondrial membrane potential ($\Delta\Psi_m$) [52–54]. Although efficient, this electron transfer process is not perfect. For instance, during the Q cycle that operates between complexes I and III, a two-step oxidation occurs in which ubiquinol is transformed into ubiquinone via an intermediary ubisemiquinone. The ubisemiquinone is capable of transferring electrons to molecular O_2, leading to the formation of O_2^- [52–54].

Organic DEP chemicals are able to interfere in the electron transfer chain in mitochondria to generate ROS [16,17,39], which includes interference by polar DEP chemicals, including redox cycling quinones such as 9,10-phenanathraquinone (see Fig. 1). We have demonstrated that this interference takes place between complexes I and III, which suggests that PM redox cycling chemicals may disrupt the Q cycle at this juncture of the electron transfer chain [39]. This disruption could favor the accumulation of ubisemiquinones, thereby contributing to $O_2^{\bullet}$ production in the mitochondria [39,55,56].

In addition to the depolarizing effect on the inner membrane, organic DEP chemicals such as quinones and PAHs can perturb the mitochondrial permeability transition (PT) pore [39]. The PT pore is a redox-, pH-, calcium-, and $\Delta\Psi_m$-dependent protein complex that plays a pivotal role in regulating mitochondrial function and controlling apoptosis in cells [57–59]. DEP chemicals lead to oxidation of vicinal thiol groups that regulate the open/closed state of the mitochondrial PT pore. This oxidation, together with PM-induced increases in intracellular free calcium, results in PT pore opening [39]. The Ca^{2+} dependence is demonstrated by the ability of cyclosporin A, an inhibitor of the Ca^{2+}-dependant chaperone, cyclophilin D, to interfere in PM-induced PT pore opening [39]. Redox cycling quinones, such as phenanathraquinone and naphthoquinone induce Ca^{2+}-dependent, cyclosporin A sensitive PT pore opening in isolated mitochondria, whereas a non–redox-cycling quinone, 9,10-anthraquinone, was inactive [39]. Large-scale PT pore opening decreases $\Delta\Psi_m$, increases $O_2^{\bullet}$ generation, releases apoptotic factors to the cytosol, disrupts ATP synthesis, and ultimately could lead to cell death [16,39,53].

Mitochondria have been shown to be a direct subcellular target for ambient UFP [8,16,39]. Ambient UFP lodge in the mitochondria of target cells such as macrophages and epithelial cells after their exposure to an aqueous suspension of UFP [8]. Morphologically, it manifests as disruption of the mitochondrial integrity, with disappearance of their cristae. Functionally, these changes are accompanied by a loss of mitochondrial membrane potential, decrease in mitochondrial mass, opening of the PT pore, ROS production, and cell death [8,39]. In contrast, fine and coarse particles do not lodge in mitochondria but can indirectly affect mitochondrial function through ROS generation and intracellular calcium flux elsewhere in the cell [8,12,34]. Why UFPs target the mitochondria is unknown.

NADPH oxidase is a membrane-assembled multi-subunit enzyme complex in phagocytic cells [60]. The holoenzyme consists of two membrane-bound (gp91^{phox} and p22^{phox}) and three cytoplasmic subunits (p40^{PHOX}, p47^{PHOX}, and p67^{PHOX}) and a small GTPase Rac1/2 [60,61]. In its unassembled form under basal cellular conditions, this enzyme is inactive. In the presence of agonists such as fMLP and opsonized zymosan, however, which interact with membrane receptors, and stimuli generated in the course of phagocytosis, NADPH oxidase is assembled and activated in the membrane [60,61]. The membrane assembly involves recruitment of the NADPH oxidase cytoplasmic subunits to the membrane, where they interact with gp91^{phox} and p22^{phox}. The catalytically active holoenzyme generates large amounts of O_2^- [60,61]. Nanosized DEP have been found to selectively damage dopaminergic neurons through the phagocytic activation of microglial NADPH oxidase and initiation of an oxidative insult [62]. This effect is decreased in cells collected from NADPH oxidase deficient (PHOX$^{-/-}$) mice and by a phagocytic inhibitor, cytochalasin D [62].

The biology of oxidative stress explains several particulate matter–induced adverse health effects

ROS are oxygen molecules that contain unpaired electrons. Fig. 5 depicts the four-electron transfer that can transform O_2 to H_2O. In the process, the addition of one, two, or three electrons can generate O_2^-, H_2O_2, and $^\bullet OH$ reactive species. ROS readily react with cellular components, such as proteins, lipids, membranes, and DNA, leading to structural damage [53,54]. ROS also can deplete cellular GSH, which leads to the accumulation of glutathione disulfide [7,17]. The accompanying decrease in the cellular GSH/glutathione disulfide ratio indicates a state of the redox disequilibrium (ie, oxidative stress) [8,17]. Oxidative stress acts as a stimulus that can initiate further cellular responses, thereby contributing to the pathogenesis of PM-induced disease.

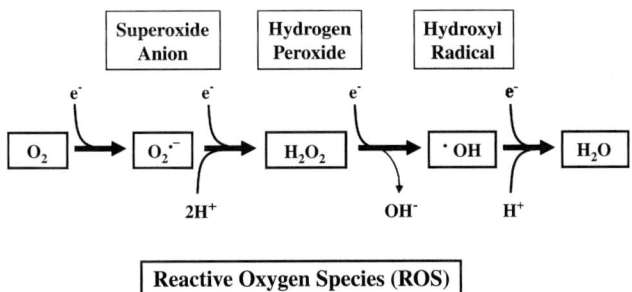

Fig. 5. ROS generation by a chain of electron acquisitions that involve the formation of superoxide, H_2O_2, the hydroxyl radical, and finally H_2O. (*Modified from* Li N, Hao M, Phalen RF, et al. Particulate air pollutants and asthma: a paradigm for the role of oxidative stress in PM-induced adverse health effects. Clin Immunol 2003;109(3):251; with permission.)

Cellular responses to oxidative stress include protective and injurious events. To explain this apparent paradox, we used biologic and proteome analyses to explore the evolving series of events in target cells, such as epithelial cells and macrophages during exposure to pro-oxidative PM chemicals [5,7,20,21,38]. This experiment led to the characterization of a hierarchical oxidative stress model (Table 3), which posits that at a lower level of oxidative stress (Tier 1), cells generate protective antioxidant and detoxification enzymes by acting on a genetic response element that requires the bZIP transcription factor, Nrf2 [7,43]. Nrf2 drives the antioxidant response element in the promoter of phase II genes, leading to the expression of antioxidant and cytoprotective enzymes [63]. Several of these phase II enzymes that have been shown to be responsive to DEP, ambient UFP, and organic DEP extracts in PM target tissue in the lung, including HO-1, glutathione-S-transferase, NADPH quinone oxidoreductase, catalase, superoxide dismutase, glutathione peroxidase, and UDP-glucoronosyltransferase [38,63]. These phase II enzymes protect against oxidative stress injury (Tiers 2 and 3), such that a reduced or compromised Tier 1 response may promote oxidant PM injury. Clinically, a compromise in Tier 1 responses can occur because of phase II enzyme polymorphisms in phase II genes or null genotypes. For instance, the glutathione-S-transferase M1 null genotype predisposes atopic people to asthma and to an enhanced allergic inflammatory response by DEP challenge in the nose [64]. Conversely, the induction of a phase II response may help people to adapt to a polluted environment and may explain why only a relatively small number of people in a population get sick when confronted with a sudden surge in ambient PM levels [63]. Adaptation can explain why repeated low-dose concentrated ambient particle exposures fail to elicit persistent lung inflammation [65].

If Tier 1 protection fails, a further increase in oxidative stress could lead to the generation of proinflammatory (Tier 2) or cytotoxic (Tier 3) effects

Table 3
Biology of oxidative stress

	Oxidative stress level Low ————————➤ High		
	Tier 1	Tier 2	Tier 3
Cellular response	Antioxidant defense	Inflammation	Toxicity
Pathways	Nrf2	NF-κB & MAPK activation	Mitochondrial perturbation (PT pore)
Biologic	Phase II antioxidant enzymes	Cytokines, chemokines, lipid peroxidation	Apoptosis, necrosis
Clinical relevance	Weakened response (susceptibility)	Asthma, adjuvant effects, atherosclerosis	? Increased ROS generation? ? epithelial shedding

(Table 3) at the cellular level. Tier 2 responses are linked to the activation of intracellular signaling pathways that impact cytokine and chemokine gene promoters [11,32,66]. An example is activation of the mitogen-activated protein kinase (MAPK) cascades [7]. These cascades are responsible for the expression and activation of AP-1 transcription factors (eg, c-Jun and c-Fos), which play a role in the transcriptional activation of proinflammatory genes, such as the genes that encod for cytokines, chemokines, and adhesion molecules. Tier 3 responses involve mitochondrial perturbation by pro-oxidative chemicals [16,18,32,43]. Although the in vivo significance of the mitochondrial pathway is uncertain, it has been demonstrated in tissue culture cells that PM interference in mitochondrial electron transfer can contribute to ROS production and the induction of apoptosis [18,32,43]. These effects can be mimicked by organic DEP extracts and redox cycling quinones and functionalized aromatic hydrocarbons present in these extracts [39].

Using the strengths of proteomics to find DEP-induced oxidative stress proteins, the principles of a hierarchical oxidative stress response could be confirmed in macrophages and epithelial cell cultures [7,32]. Two-dimensional gel electrophoresis demonstrated the appearance of >50 newly expressed proteins, which could be subtracted from the expression profile by pretreatment of the cells with NAC [7]. At the lowest tier of oxidative stress (Tier 1), the expression of catalase, superoxide dismutase, and HO-1 confirm the involvement of Nrf2-regulated enzymes that play a role in the suppression of inflammation through their antioxidant activities [63,66]. This finding was confirmed by showing that DEPs and UFPs increase the accumulation of Nrf2 in the nucleus, including their ability to activate the antioxidant response element [63]. The Nrf2 translocation to the nucleus depends on a prolongation of the half-life of this transcription factor by interference in its proteasomal degradation [63]. Under basal conditions, Nrf2 exhibits a short (approximately 15-minute) half-life because it is continuously being shuttled to the 20S proteosome by a chaperone, Keap-1 [63]. In the presence of electrophilic chemicals, Nrf2 uncouples from Keap-1, which leads to its withdrawal from the proteasomal degradation pathway and the accumulation in the cell and the nucleus [63,67]. Phosphoproteome analysis performed in parallel with cytokine array has confirmed that activation of the ERK, p38, and Jun kinase cascades are linked to the induction of proinflammatory responses [32].

Each tier of oxidative stress is sensitive to the effects of the thiol antioxidant, NAC [7,16,18]. NAC is capable of quenching oxygen radicals and acting as a precursor to GSH synthesis [7,16]. NAC is capable of covalent modification of electrophilic chemicals and cellular proteins [7]. These interactions prevent redox cycling of organic PM chemicals and can protect key cellular cysteine residues against oxidative cross-linking. It is possible, therefore, that low levels of oxidative stress may target NAC-protected cysteines that are involved in the binding of Nrf2 to Keap-1 [63]. Similarly, at Tiers 2 and 3 of the hierarchical oxidative stress response, it is possible that NAC may protect SH groups that are involved in the inactivation of mitogen-activated protein kinase phosphatases or in the opening of the mitochondrial PT pore [7]. A possible unifying hypothesis to explain the hierarchical response is that the cysteines that regulate each of these tiers are differentially sensitive to oxidative modification by ROS or electrophilic chemicals.

A key question is whether the hierarchical oxidative stress model is relevant to in vivo disease outcomes in PM-exposed people. Although it is difficult to envisage a large-scale oxidative stress response that targets an entire organ or the intact body, it is probably more practical to think of the tiered response as a dynamic equilibrium between pro-oxidant and antioxidant forces at the level of specific tissue targets. For instance, in an individual who has asthma and suffers from low-grade airway inflammation, a sudden surge in ambient PM levels could increase particle deposition at airway bifurcation points. These so-called "hot spots" of deposition are richly endowed with bronchial epithelial cells, macrophages, and immune cells, such as antigen-presenting cells and lymphocytes [68]. The ability of the epithelium, macrophages, and antigen-presenting cells to mount a phase II response may prevent or suppress a potential chain of immune activating events that can culminate in IgE switching in B cells because of functional changes in helper T lymphocytes [20]. The converse also may be true, however; namely, that abundant ROS generation that pushes the local tissue response to Tier 2 may perturb antigen-presenting cell activity and immune activation to complete the IgE switch. At this point, the committed response of memory T cells and B cells could transfer the immune response to the entire respiratory mucosa. A focal area in which proinflammatory dominate anti-inflammatory responses may lead to more generalized effects. Similar scenarios can be envisaged in the pathophysiology of an atherosclerotic plaque, in which pro- and antioxidative influences may determine whether lipid-laden macrophages undergo apoptosis or whether the overlying endothelium may express adhesion molecules that favor platelet adhesion and thrombus formation. Both events contribute to fatal heart attacks, which are epidemiologically associated with a sudden rise in ambient PM levels [15].

The importance of oxidative stress in future research and therapy for particulate matter–induced adverse health effects

The recognition of the role of oxidative stress in PM-induced adverse health effects is an important cornerstone for future research. First, it is important to characterize all the chemical components that play a role in ROS generation for toxicologic and regulatory purposes. If PAH and quinone analyses prove to be accurate predictors of adverse health effects, it may be important to monitor these substances in ambient air. In this regard, the high PAH content of UFPs collected in the Los Angeles basin has been shown to be a good predictor of the ability of these particles to generate oxidative stress in macrophages and epithelial cells [8]. Even if PAHs are not directly responsible for ROS generation, their assessment could serve as a proxy for redox cycling chemicals that are responsible for adverse health effects. Second, the recognition that particle size and reactive surface area play an important role in predicting pro-oxidative particle effects could mean that in addition to a mass standard, particle number and surface area may need to be incorporated into the regulatory assessments. This addition could be of considerable importance in following PM effects in areas in which vehicular traffic is a major contributor to ambient PM levels, especially as it pertains to UFP levels. A third consideration is the development of in vivo markers for oxidative stress that can be used to look for subclinical PM responses. This consideration is particularly important for dissecting the apparent disconnect between macroscale epidemiology, which shows considerable morbidity and mortality caused by ambient PM exposure, and smaller scale exposure studies, which often fail to show significant health effects. A possible explanation is that only a small percentage (eg, 1%–2%) of individuals is truly sensitive to PM and more likely to be excluded on a chance basis when selections are made for human exposure studies. To identify susceptible individuals, it is important to develop in vivo oxidative stress markers that can be used to identify susceptible people for study purposes.

Understanding of the role of oxidative stress in disease pathogenesis is also important from a therapy perspective. Based on our principal hypotheses, namely that (1) oxidative stress is a key mechanism by which PM impacts allergic inflammation and asthma exacerbation and (2) Nrf2-mediated antioxidant defense protects against the proinflammatory effects of PM, we predict that therapeutic interventions that lead to phase II enzyme expression could provide a novel treatment approach for asthma. Although several types of antioxidants have been tried in patients who have asthma [69–71], there is no clear consensus that antioxidant therapy is useful in this disease. In our opinion, previous attempts have been hampered by the lack of appreciation that certain asthmatic subsets (eg, atopic subjects with a glutathione-S-transferase M1 null genotype [64]) may be more prone to the adverse biologic effects of oxidative stress. There may be a lack of appreciation of the redundancy of oxidative stress pathways once ROS production is already in progress. Initial sources of ROS production could be redox cycling and electrophilic chemicals, which generate ROS through spontaneous particle-mediated and enzymatic reactions. This could yield to or be overtaken by additional sources of ROS once tissue inflammation is involved. We propose that interference in oxidative stress must commence before the initial ROS production by pro-oxidative chemicals to be effective and prevent the redundant mechanisms that operate once radical production is in place. Increased expression of phase II enzymes is an attractive candidate to accomplish the goal of interfering in lung and heart diseases. Based on the detoxification and antioxidant effects of phase II enzymes, they could be effective in neutralizing the adverse biologic effects of redox cycling organic chemicals by scavenging a wide range of ROS and detoxifying the inducing chemicals [63]. Phase II enzymes also enhance GSH synthesis and specialize in the removal of a wide range of ROS [63].

Phase II enzyme expression can be achieved by oral administration of two chemical compounds, α-lipoic acid (αLA) [72–74] and sulforaphane [75]. Both compounds function through Nrf2 release and antioxidant response element activation. αLA is a disulfide derivative of octanoic acid that forms an intracellular disulfide bond in its oxidized form. High electron density that results from special positioning of the two sulfur atoms in the 1,2-dithiolane ring allows αLA to reduce redox-sensitive molecules. αLA in its reduced form (DHLA) is a strong reductant that is more easily oxidized than monothiols. Exogenously supplied αLA is absorbed, transported to tissues, and reduced to DHLA. αLA and DHLA are highly reactive against various ROS in vitro. αLA and DHLA redox also are capable of regenerating GSH. This action includes Nrf2-mediated expression of γ-glutamylcysteine ligase, the rate-limiting enzyme in GSH synthesis [73]. In a murine asthma model, αLA treatment significantly reduced airway hyperreactivity, BAL eosinophilia, and airway inflammation [74]. Sulforaphane is a chemical found in foods such as broccoli and is capable of inducing various phase II enzymes, which results in the enhancement of cellular antioxidant capacity [75]. Sulforaphane induces phase II enzyme expression by uncoupling Nrf2 from its chaperone, Keap-I, and allowing the transcription factor to accumulate in the nucleus [63,75].

Summary

Numerous reports have linked oxidative stress to PM-induced adverse health effects. ROS production is related to redox cycling organic chemicals and transition metals bound to the PM surface and may originate from the particle surface and enzymatically catalyzed reactions in target cells. UFPs are more toxic than larger ambient particles in the Los Angeles basin, based on their ability to generate ROS. The PM-induced oxidative stress response at cellular level is a hierarchical event. Oxidative stress responses range from protective phase II enzyme expression, at low levels of oxidative stress, to activation of proinflammatory signaling pathways at higher levels of oxidative stress. This dynamic equilibrium may determine who responds to PM, what type of response is generated, and who could benefit from rational antioxidant therapy that leads to increased phase II enzyme expression.

References

[1] National Academy of Science National Research Council. Research priorities for airborne particulate matter: I. Immediate priorities and a long-range Research Portfolio. Washington, DC: National Academy of Science National Research Council; 1998.

[2] Nel AE, Diaz-Sanchez D, Ng D, et al. Enhancement of allergic inflammation by the interaction between diesel exhaust particles and the immune system. J Allergy Clin Immunol 1998; 102(4 Pt 1):539–54.

[3] Ghio AJ, Devlin RB. Inflammatory lung injury after bronchial instillation of air pollution particles. Am J Respir Crit Care Med 2001;164(4):704–8.

[4] Muranaka M, Suzuki S, Koizumi K, et al. Adjuvant activity of diesel-exhaust particulates for the production of IgE antibody in mice. J Allergy Clin Immunol 1986;77(4):616–23.

[5] Gurgueira SA, Lawrence J, Coull B, et al. Rapid increases in the steady-state concentration of reactive oxygen species in the lungs and heart after particulate air pollution inhalation. Environ Health Perspect 2002;110(8):749–55.

[6] Lim HB, Ichinose T, Miyabara Y, et al. Involvement of superoxide and nitric oxide on airway inflammation and hyperresponsiveness induced by diesel exhaust particles in mice. Free Radic Biol Med 1998;25(6):635–44.

[7] Xiao GG, Wang M, Li N, Loo JA, et al. Use of proteomics to demonstrate a hierarchical oxidative stress response to diesel exhaust particle chemicals in a macrophage cell line. J Biol Chem 2003;278(50):50781–90.

[8] Li N, Sioutas C, Cho A, et al. Ultrafine particulate pollutants induce oxidative stress and mitochondrial damage. Environ Health Perspect 2003;111(4):455–60.

[9] Silbajoris R, Ghio AJ, Samet JM, et al. In vivo and in vitro correlation of pulmonary MAP kinase activation following metallic exposure. Inhal Toxicol 2000;12(6):453–68.

[10] Donaldson K, Tran CL. Inflammation caused by particles and fibers. Inhal Toxicol 2002; 14(1):5–27.

[11] Nel AE, az-Sanchez D, Li N. The role of particulate pollutants in pulmonary inflammation and asthma: evidence for the involvement of organic chemicals and oxidative stress. Curr Opin Pulm Med 2001;7(1):20–6.

[12] Nel A. Atmosphere: air pollution-related illness: effects of particles. Science 2005;308(5723): 804–6.

[13] Samet JM, Dominici F, Curriero FC, et al. Fine particulate air pollution and mortality in 20 US cities, 1987–1994. N Engl J Med 2000;343(24):1742–9.

[14] Dockery DW, Pope CA III, Xu X, et al. An association between air pollution and mortality in six US cities. N Engl J Med 1993;329(24):1753–9.

[15] Brook RD, Franklin B, Cascio W, et al. Air pollution and cardiovascular disease: a statement for healthcare professionals from the Expert Panel on Population and Prevention Science of the American Heart Association. Circulation 2004;109(21):2655–71.

[16] Hiura TS, Li N, Kaplan R, et al. The role of a mitochondrial pathway in the induction of apoptosis by chemicals extracted from diesel exhaust particles. J Immunol 2000;165(5): 2703–11.

[17] Li N, Wang M, Oberley TD, et al. Comparison of the pro-oxidative and proinflammatory effects of organic diesel exhaust particle chemicals in bronchial epithelial cells and macrophages. J Immunol 2002;169(8):4531–41.

[18] Hiura TS, Kaszubowski MP, Li N, et al. Chemicals in diesel exhaust particles generate reactive oxygen radicals and induce apoptosis in macrophages. J Immunol 1999;163(10): 5582–91.

[19] Kumagai Y, Arimoto T, Shinyashiki M, et al. Generation of reactive oxygen species during interaction of diesel exhaust particle components with NADPH-cytochrome P450 reductase and involvement of the bioactivation in the DNA damage. Free Radic Biol Med 1997;22(3): 479–87.

[20] Whitekus MJ, Li N, Zhang M, et al. Thiol antioxidants inhibit the adjuvant effects of aerosolized diesel exhaust particles in a murine model for ovalbumin sensitization. J Immunol 2002;168(5):2560–7.

[21] Rhoden CR, Lawrence J, Godleski JJ, et al. N-acetylcysteine prevents lung inflammation after short-term inhalation exposure to concentrated ambient particles. Toxicol Sci 2004; 79(2):296–303.

[22] Rhoden CR, Wellenius GA, Ghelfi E, et al. PM-induced cardiac oxidative stress and dysfunction are mediated by autonomic stimulation. Biochim Biophys Acta 2005;1725(3): 305–13.

[23] Knaapen AM, Shi T, Borm PJ, et al. Soluble metals as well as the insoluble particle fraction are involved in cellular DNA damage induced by particulate matter. Mol Cell Biochem 2002; 234–235(1–2):317–26.

[24] Arimoto T, Kadiiska MB, Sato K, et al. Synergistic production of lung free radicals by diesel exhaust particles and endotoxin. Am J Respir Crit Care Med 2005;171(4):379–87.

[25] Sanbongi C, Takano H, Osakabe N, et al. Rosmarinic acid inhibits lung injury induced by diesel exhaust particles. Free Radic Biol Med 2003;34(8):1060–9.

[26] Nabeyrat E, Jones GE, Fenwick PS, et al. Mitogen-activated protein kinases mediate peroxynitrite-induced cell death in human bronchial epithelial cells. Am J Physiol Lung Cell Mol Physiol 2003;284(6):L1112–20.

[27] Nightingale JA, Maggs R, Cullinan P, et al. Airway inflammation after controlled exposure to diesel exhaust particulates. Am J Respir Crit Care Med 2000;162(1):161–6.

[28] Abraham NG, Kappas A. Heme oxygenase and the cardiovascular-renal system. Free Radic Biol Med 2005;39(1):1–25.

[29] Silkoff PE. Noninvasive measurement of airway inflammation using exhaled nitric oxide and induced sputum: current status and future use. Clin Chest Med 2000;21(2): 345–60.

[30] Steerenberg PA, Nierkens S, Fischer PH, et al. Traffic-related air pollution affects peak expiratory flow, exhaled nitric oxide, and inflammatory nasal markers. Arch Environ Health 2001;56(2):167–74.

[31] van Amsterdam JG, Verlaan BP, van Loveren H, et al. Air pollution is associated with increased level of exhaled nitric oxide in nonsmoking healthy subjects. Arch Environ Health 1999;54(5):331–5.

[32] Wang M, Xiao GG, Li N, et al. Use of a fluorescent phosphoprotein dye to characterize oxidative stress-induced signaling pathway components in macrophage and epithelial cultures exposed to diesel exhaust particle chemicals. Electrophoresis 2005;26(11): 2092–108.

[33] Cho AK, Sioutas C, Miguel AH, et al. Redox activity of airborne particulate matter at different sites in the Los Angeles Basin. Environ Res 2005;99(1):40–7.

[34] Donaldson K, Stone V, Borm PJ, et al. Oxidative stress and calcium signaling in the adverse effects of environmental particles (PM10). Free Radic Biol Med 2003;34(11): 1369–82.

[35] Carter JD, Ghio AJ, Samet JM, et al. Cytokine production by human airway epithelial cells after exposure to an air pollution particle is metal-dependent. Toxicol Appl Pharmacol 1997; 146(2):180–8.

[36] Lay JC, Bennett WD, Kim CS, et al. Retention and intracellular distribution of instilled iron oxide particles in human alveolar macrophages. Am J Respir Cell Mol Biol 1998;18(5): 687–95.

[37] Ghio AJ, Hall A, Bassett MA, et al. Exposure to concentrated ambient air particles alters hematologic indices in humans. Inhal Toxicol 2003;15(14):1465–78.

[38] Li N, Venkatesan MI, Miguel A, et al. Induction of heme oxygenase-1 expression in macrophages by diesel exhaust particle chemicals and quinones via the antioxidant-responsive element. J Immunol 2000;165(6):3393–401.

[39] Xia T, Korge P, Weiss JN, et al. Quinones and aromatic chemical compounds in particulate matter induce mitochondrial dysfunction: implications for ultrafine particle toxicity. Environ Health Perspect 2004;112(14):1347–58.

[40] Penning TM, Burczynski ME, Hung CF, et al. Dihydrodiol dehydrogenases and polycyclic aromatic hydrocarbon activation: generation of reactive and redox active o-quinones. Chem Res Toxicol 1999;12(1):1–18.

[41] Baulig A, Garlatti M, Bonvallot V, et al. Involvement of reactive oxygen species in the metabolic pathways triggered by diesel exhaust particles in human airway epithelial cells. Am J Physiol Lung Cell Mol Physiol 2003;285(3):L671–9.

[42] Seagrave J, Gigliotti A, McDonald JD, et al. Composition, toxicity, and mutagenicity of particulate and semivolatile emissions from heavy-duty compressed natural gas-powered vehicles. Toxicol Sci 2005;87(1):232–41.

[43] Li N, Kim S, Wang M, et al. Use of a stratified oxidative stress model to study the biological effects of ambient concentrated and diesel exhaust particulate matter. Inhal Toxicol 2002; 14(5):459–86.

[44] Farmer PB, Singh R, Kaur B, et al. Molecular epidemiology studies of carcinogenic environmental pollutants: effects of polycyclic aromatic hydrocarbons (PAHs) in environmental pollution on exogenous and oxidative DNA damage. Mutat Res 2003;544(2–3):397–402.

[45] Perera FP, Jedrychowski W, Rauh V, et al. Molecular epidemiologic research on the effects of environmental pollutants on the fetus. Environ Health Perspect 1999;107(Suppl 3):451–60.

[46] Dejmek J, Solansky I, Benes I, et al. The impact of polycyclic aromatic hydrocarbons and fine particles on pregnancy outcome. Environ Health Perspect 2000;108(12):1159–64.

[47] Donaldson K, Stone V. Current hypotheses on the mechanisms of toxicity of ultrafine particles. Ann Ist Super Sanita 2003;39(3):405–10.

[48] Oberdörster G, Oberdörster E, Oberdörster J. Nanotoxicology: an emerging discipline evolving from studies of ultrafine particles. Environ Health Perspect 2005;113(7):823–39.

[49] Pan CJ, Schmitz DA, Cho AK, et al. Inherent redox properties of diesel exhaust particles: catalysis of the generation of reactive oxygen species by biological reductants. Toxicol Sci 2004;81(1):225–32.

[50] Valavanidis A, Fiotakis K, Bakeas E, et al. Electron paramagnetic resonance study of the generation of reactive oxygen species catalysed by transition metals and quinoid redox cycling by inhalable ambient particulate matter. Redox Rep 2005;10(1):37–51.

[51] Sagai M, Saito H, Ichinose T, et al. Biological effects of diesel exhaust particles. I. In vitro production of superoxide and in vivo toxicity in mouse. Free Radic Biol Med 1993;14(1): 37–47.

[52] Andreyev AY, Kushnareva YE, Starkov AA. Mitochondrial metabolism of reactive oxygen species. Biochemistry (Mosc) 2005;70(2):200–14.

[53] Papa S, Skulachev VP. Reactive oxygen species, mitochondria, apoptosis and aging. Mol Cell Biochem 1997;174(1–2):305–19.

[54] Raha S, Robinson BH. Mitochondria, oxygen free radicals, disease and ageing. Trends Biochem Sci 2000;25(10):502–8.

[55] Walter L, Nogueira V, Leverve X, et al. Three classes of ubiquinone analogs regulate the mitochondrial permeability transition pore through a common site. J Biol Chem 2000;275(38): 29521–7.

[56] Fontaine E, Ichas F, Bernardi P. A ubiquinone-binding site regulates the mitochondrial permeability transition pore. J Biol Chem 1998;273(40):25734–40.

[57] Zamzami N, Kroemer G. The mitochondrion in apoptosis: how Pandora's Box opens. Nat Rev Mol Cell Biol 2001;2:67–71.

[58] Halestrap AP, McStay GP, Clarke SJ. The permeability transition pore complex: another view. Biochimie 2002;84(2–3):153–66.

[59] Bernardi P, Petronilli V, Di Lisa F, et al. A mitochondrial perspective on cell death. Trends Biochem Sci 2001;26(2):112–7.

[60] Babior BM. NADPH oxidase. Curr Opin Immunol 2004;16(1):42–7.

[61] Brandes RP, Kreuzer J. Vascular NADPH oxidases: molecular mechanisms of activation. Cardiovasc Res 2005;65(1):16–27.

[62] Block ML, Wu X, Pei Z, et al. Nanometer size diesel exhaust particles are selectively toxic to dopaminergic neurons: the role of microglia, phagocytosis, and NADPH oxidase. FASEB J 2004;18(13):1618–20.

[63] Li N, Alam J, Venkatesan MI, et al. Nrf2 is a key transcription factor that regulates antiox-idant defense in macrophages and epithelial cells: protecting against the proinflammatory and oxidizing effects of diesel exhaust chemicals. J Immunol 2004;173(5):3467–81.

[64] Fryer A, Bianco A, Hepple M, et al. Polymorphism at the glutathione S-transferase GSTP1 locus: a new marker for bronchial hyperresponsiveness and asthma. Am J Respir Crit Care Med 2000;161(5):1437–42.

[65] Lippmann M, Gordon T, Chen LC. Effects of subchronic exposures to concentrated ambient particles (CAPs) in mice. I. Introduction, objectives, and experimental plan. Inhal Toxicol 2005;17(4–5):177–87.

[66] Li N, Hao M, Phalen RF, et al. Particulate air pollutants and asthma: a paradigm for the role of oxidative stress in PM-induced adverse health effects. Clin Immunol 2003;109(3):250–65.

[67] Zhang DD, Hannink M. Distinct cysteine residues in Keap1 are required for Keap1-dependent ubiquitination of Nrf2 and for stabilization of Nrf2 by chemopreventive agents and oxidative stress. Mol Cell Biol 2003;23(22):8137–51.

[68] Hao M, Comier S, Wang M, et al. Diesel exhaust particles exert acute effects on airway in-flammation and function in murine allergen provocation models. J Allergy Clin Immunol 2003;112(5):905–14.

[69] Bylin G, Hedenstierna G, Lagerstrand L, et al. No influence of acetylcysteine on gas exchange and spirometry in chronic asthma. Eur J Respir Dis 1987;71(2):102–7.

[70] Pearson PJK, Lewis SA, Britton J, et al. Vitamin E supplements in asthma: a parallel group randomised placebo controlled trial. Thorax 2004;59(8):652–6.

[71] Ram FS, Rowe BH, Kaur B. Vitamin C supplementation for asthma. Cochrane Database Syst Rev 2004;3:CD000993.

[72] Flier J, Van Muiswinkel FL, Jongenelen CA, et al. The neuroprotective antioxidant alpha-lipoic acid induces detoxication enzymes in cultured astroglial cells. Free Radic Res 2002; 36(6):695–9.

[73] Suh JH, Shenvi SV, Dixon BM, et al. Decline in transcriptional activity of Nrf2 causes age-related loss of glutathione synthesis, which is reversible with lipoic acid. Proc Natl Acad Sci U S A 2004;101(10):3381–6.

[74] Sook Cho Y, Lee J, Lee TH, et al. α-Lipoic acid inhibits airway inflammation and hyperres-ponsiveness in a mouse model of asthma. J Allergy Clin Immunol 2004;114(2):429–35.

[75] Lee JS, Surh YJ. Nrf2 as a novel molecular target for chemoprevention. Cancer Lett 2005; 224(2):171–84.

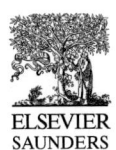
ELSEVIER
SAUNDERS

Clin Occup Environ Med
5 (4) 837–848

CLINICS IN
OCCUPATIONAL AND
ENVIRONMENTAL
MEDICINE

Long-Term Effects of Exposure to Particulate Air Pollution

Joel Schwartz, PhD

*Department of Environmental Health, Harvard School of Public Health, Landmark Center,
Room 415L West, 401 Park Drive, PO Box 15677, Boston, MA 02215, USA*

In the twelfth century, Maimonides said:

> "Comparing the air of cities to the air of deserts and arid lands is like comparing waters that are befouled and turbid to waters that are fine and pure. In the city, because of the height of its buildings, the narrowness of its streets, and all that pours forth from its inhabitants …the air becomes stagnant, turbid, thick, misty and foggy… If there is no choice in this matter, for we have grown up in cities and have become accustomed to them, you should select from the cities one of open horizons… endeavor to at least dwell at the outskirts of the city." [1]

Maimonides, of course, was referring to smoke: particulate air pollution. Since the twelfth century, considerable work has been done to elucidate the effects of turbid air. Most of that research has studied acute effects of particles. Although studies of longer term exposure are more difficult, expensive, and rarer, they provide deeper insights into the ultimate burden of exposure. These studies suggest that the effects of longer term exposures are more than just the daily sum of the acute effects. Because most of the studies of acute effects have examined changes in health status occurring within days of the exposure, this article takes a broad definition of long-term exposure to include averaging times of months to years. The advantage of this approach is that it allows us to ask how the answers to our questions about the health effects of exposure to airborne particulate matter (PM) change as we change the averaging times.

Respiratory effects

Lung function

A seminal early study that associated long-term exposure to particles with adverse health effects examined the lung function of British postal

E-mail address: joel@hsph.harvard.edu

1526-0046/06/$ - see front matter © 2006 Elsevier Inc. All rights reserved.
doi:10.1016/j.coem.2006.07.008

workers and found that workers in large urban areas with higher smoke concentrations consistently had lower lung function. The advantage of this study was that the postal workers generally stayed in the same counties all of their careers and were of the same social status. Subsequent studies have examined the association of lung function in adults and children with long-term exposure to particles.

Using data from the first National Health and Nutrition Examination Survey, Chestnut and colleagues [2] found that total suspended PM was associated with lower lung function in the United States. The Swiss Study on Air Pollution and Lung Disease in Adults (SAPALDIA) collected questionnaire data, pulmonary function data, and air pollution measurements in a random sample of eight communities in Switzerland and reported a strong association between particles smaller than 10 μM in aerodynamic diameter and adult lung function [3]. More recently, a study of adult women resident in their district of Tokyo for 8 years found that pulmonary function decline over the period increased in a dose-dependent manner with the concentration of particles in their district [4]. Lubinski and coworkers [5] examined lung function in healthy nonsmoking young men in Poland and reported decreases in the FEV_1/FVC ratio, and FEV_1 as a percent of predicted was associated with increased exposure to particles.

Other studies have examined the impacts of particles in children. In the 1980s, Schwartz [6] reported that pulmonary function was decreased with increasing exposure to particles in 6- to 18-year old individuals, using data from the Second National Health and Nutrition Examination Survey(NHANES II). The 24-city study examined lung function and air pollution concentrations in US and Canadian towns that were chosen to allow better differentiation between particles, acid particles, and ozone. Raizenne and coworkers [7] reported that $PM_{2.5}$ and acid aerosols were associated with pulmonary function decrements in that cross-sectional study. The Southern California Children's Health Study has been following several cohorts of children for more than a decade and has produced a substantial body of work on the impact of air pollution on children's respiratory health. This study has allowed a longitudinal—as opposed to a cross-sectional—assessment of the associations. Most recently, Gauderman and coworkers [8] reported that exposure to $PM_{2.5}$ was associated with decrements of lung function growth between 10 and 18 years of age. This decrement was even more strongly associated with elemental carbon level, a marker for traffic particles. Similarly, Horak and coworkers [9] followed Austrian schoolchildren over a 3-year period and found that after adjustment for covariates, including initial lung function, lung function growth rates were associated with PM_{10} exposure.

Respiratory symptoms

Long-term exposure to particles also has been associated with respiratory symptoms. Dockery and coworkers [10] compared symptom reports of children across six communities in the eastern United States with varying levels of pollution and found that chronic bronchitis and chest illnesses in children were associated with exposure to particulate air pollution. No association was seen with asthma or wheezing. Subsequent studies in the United States and Europe confirmed that particulate exposure (across communities) was associated with higher rates of chronic cough and bronchitis symptoms in children and the lack of association with wheezing and asthma. For example, a large study ($n = 4470$) examined school children in ten communities in Switzerland and reported an odds ratio for bronchitis of 2.88 (95% CI 1.69–4.89) for PM_{10} exposure between the most and least polluted community [11]. The previously mentioned Southern California study examined 3676 children across 12 communities and found that bronchitis was associated with PM_{10}, but only among children with asthma [12]. The largest study was the 24-city study, which examined 13,369 children [13]. Particulate air pollution was associated with bronchitis episodes across these communities.

Although comparisons across communities have demonstrated associations between PM levels and bronchitic symptoms, comparisons of exposures to traffic related particles within communities have begun to report associations with asthma. For example, Lin and coworkers [14] geocoded the residential addresses of children admitted to the hospital in Erie County, New York (excluding Buffalo) for asthma and age-matched controls admitted for nonrespiratory conditions. This information was linked to data on vehicle miles traveled on their street. The odds of asthma (adjusted for poverty level) for living within 200 meters of a street with the highest tertile of traffic density was 1.93 (95% CI 1.13, 3.29), and children who had asthma were more likely to have truck traffic on their street. Another study analyzed data from two birth cohorts totaling 1756 children in Munich [15]. Geographic information system modeling was used to estimate the concentrations of traffic related particles and NO_2 outside the birth addresses of all of the children. These pollutants were associated with dry cough at night in the first year of life. Brauer and coworkers [16] examined a birth cohort of approximately 4000 children in the Netherlands and found that traffic-related pollution was associated with increased risk of wheeze and physician-diagnosed asthma. A case control study of 6147 children in Nottingham, England found increased risk of wheeze associated with living within 90 meters of a roadway [17]. Although some studies showed no increased risk, the overwhelming weight of the recent evidence suggests that traffic pollution is associated with the risk of developing asthma [18].

Lending some credence to these reports is the study by Giroux and coworkers [19], who contrasted exhaled NO in children who had asthma and were living in urban areas with children staying in a national park in the mountains. They found that the exhaled NO concentrations in the urban children who had asthma were more than double the levels in the children who had asthma who were staying in the national park, which suggests that urban air pollution is associated with pulmonary inflammation.

Long-term exposure to PM also has been associated with the development of chronic respiratory symptoms in adults. For example, Schwartz [20] reported in 1993 that chronic pulmonary symptoms, such as bronchitis, were associated with long-term exposure to air pollution in the NHANES II study adults. Using data from the Seventh Day Adventist Study, several papers have reported associations between particle exposure and chronic respiratory symptoms, mostly recently using $PM_{2.5}$ as the exposure [21]. Avino and coworkers [22] also reported an association in a more limited two-community study. An interesting case control study by Karakatsani [23] used in home examinations by physicians included pulmonary function testing to confirm self-reports of chronic respiratory conditions in adults and in age- and gender-matched controls. A geographic model was used to assign individual exposure values, which were associated with the risk of chronic bronchitis and chronic obstructive pulmonary disease.

Mortality

Although episode studies since the Meuse Valley disaster of 1930 indicated that PM could increase death rates and time series studies in the late 1980s and early 1990s confirmed that these associations persisted at concentrations below then-current air quality standards, these studies left unclear the extent to which mortality was displaced [24]. In particular, if the air pollution–associated deaths were occurring only a few days to weeks early, then one would expect little difference in life expectancy between locations with higher versus lower pollution concentrations. One also would not assign great public health significance to the early deaths.

One early sign that this was not the case came from the London Smog disaster of December 1952 [25]. The air quality returned to baseline levels within 5 days. If the great increase in deaths that occurred in that episode (in inner London, the death rate quadrupled) were merely borrowed from the next week or two, then one would have expected fewer deaths in those weeks. Instead, as shown in Fig. 1, the death rate declined more slowly than the pollution levels and did not return to baseline, let alone below baseline, in the subsequent month. A recent reanalysis has suggested that total deaths attributable to the episode were as much as three times the original estimates [26]. This result is consistent with the view that increased PM concentrations did not deplete the frail pool of subjects with substantial likelihood of dying shortly but rather increased recruitment into it, which resulted in a more sustained increase in mortality [27]. This issue is discussed in greater detail later in the article.

The first evidence that there was an effect of long-term mortality on life expectancy came from early cross-sectional ecologic studies that compared age-adjusted (or age/race/sex-adjusted) mortality rates and long-term average air pollution concentrations in US cities [28]. These studies consistently indicated that higher air pollution communities had higher death rates,

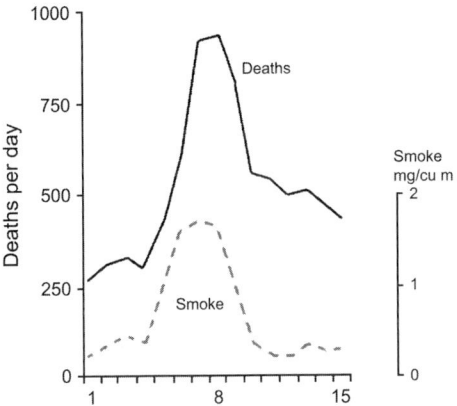

Fig. 1. Daily deaths and daily average black smoke concentrations in London in December 1952.

although the high correlation between particles and SO_2 concentrations across cities in the 1970s made it difficult to distinguish between the two pollutants [29]. These studies used ecologic data on the community level for cigarette sales, income, and other potential confounders to control for any such confounding factors, but the ecologic nature of the data resulted in little emphasis being given to them in health risk assessments.

Stronger evidence came with the arrival of prospective cohort studies. The Harvard Six City Study provided the first clear evidence that particles did reduce life expectancy and that the effect was predominantly with $PM_{2.5}$ and not with coarse particles (particles with diameters between 2.5 and 10 μM) [30]. Equally importantly, the Six City Study showed no evidence of confounding by any of the covariates examined except age. Because the earlier cross-sectional analyses had used age-adjusted death rates, it suggested that they were unlikely to have been confounded. This study followed a cohort of subjects randomly recruited from specific neighborhoods in six US cities that were chosen to represent a range of exposures to particles and sulfur oxides. Monitoring was conducted by the study investigators at locations central to the neighborhoods in which participants lived.

This association was confirmed by the American Cancer Society (ACS) Study. That study, which covered 150 cities across the United States (essentially all cities in the country), also showed significant associations between $PM_{2.5}$ and SO_4^{-2} concentrations and life expectancy [31]. In contrast to the Six City Study, the ACS study participants represented a convenience sample recruited by volunteers of the ACS from among their neighbors. Although there was no selection of cities based on pollution concentrations, essentially all US cities with populations more than 250,000 were included. Air monitoring was obtained from the US Environmental Protection Agency's inhalable particle network and from sulfate measurements taken from particle filters from routinely collected state monitoring. Monitors could be anywhere in the metropolitan statistical area, including in different counties, and often were distant from the homes of the participants. Although the ACS study found a significant association between PM2.5 and SO_4^{-2} and life expectancy, the magnitude of the risk was lower than in the Six City Study. Examination of that study for confounding found little evidence for it and suggested that the earlier cross-sectional studies were valid.

Subsequent analyses of both cohorts have extended the mortality follow-up period and confirmed the basic associations and the differences in slope [32]. Of particular interest is a more recent study from the Netherlands. Hoek and colleagues [33] reported the results of a cohort study from that country. In this cohort, geostatistical regression models were fit to estimate exposure to particles at each participant's home address. In that study, a substantially greater coefficient was found.

Because the relative ranking of the quality of the exposure assessment for these three studies is the same as the relative ranking of the slope estimates, it suggests that the lower slopes are the result of measurement error and the higher slope is the more appropriate one. Further support for this hypothesis comes from a recent reanalysis of the ACS study that only used monitors in the same county of residence of each subject to assign exposure. That study found a higher coefficient for the effects of sulfate particles on mortality than the original study [34]. Even more intriguingly, a recent study examined only the 22,905 participants of the ACS study living in Southern California using a geographic information system (GIS)-based exposure model, they reported even larger effect size estimates for $PM_{2.5}$, which approached those of the Dutch cohort [35]. The observation across five cohorts that more detailed geographic-based exposure results in greater risk estimates suggests that current risk assessments, which are usually based on the ACS study, may be substantially underestimating the impact of particles.

Several other studies also have added to the weight of evidence linking particle concentrations in the air to life expectancy. For example, a 25-year follow-up of the French air pollution and chronic respiratory diseases (PAARC) study recently reported associations between survival in the cohort and neighborhood level concentrations of particles [36]. The Seventh Day Adventist cohort also reported an association between $PM_{2.5}$ and all-cause mortality [37]. Given the strong evidence in the cohort studies that the cross-sectional ecologic studies are not confounded, it is noteworthy that two new such studies have reported an association between GIS-coded census-tract level particle exposures and stroke [38] and between metropolitan statistical area-level PM_{10} concentrations and hospitalization of the elderly [39].

Reversibility

Recently, studies have begun to examine whether chronic effects of long-term exposure to air pollution are reversed if the exposure is reduced. This finding is important for several reasons. First, it is more convincing epidemiologically. Different towns differ in many regards, and although these studies attempt to control for confounding by measuring individual risk factors, they are always subject to the concern that they may have missed one that confounds the air pollution association. If the prevalence rates change within town as the air pollution changes and those changes fit on the same dose-response curve as the original cross-sectional association, this information provides great assurance that the association is not confounded, because the factors that are likely to confound an association of temporal change are usually different from those that might confound a cross-sectional study. These studies of temporal trend are also important for health impact assessment. If the effects of long-term exposure take many years to develop, one might have to wait many years after a reduction in air quality to see improvements in health. Evidence that this is not the case suggests that improvements in air quality will be followed quickly by improvements in health. This finding is particularly important when cost-benefit analyses are performed to evaluate environmental regulations, because benefits that occur in the distant future are usually discounted to reflect that preventing a case currently is of greater value than preventing a case in 10 years. Finally, if long-term exposure is not all that long after all, then we should begin to see some correspondence between such studies and time series studies that start to lengthen the exposure period examined. Recent work suggests that the last point is a fruitful area of investigation.

A recent study that examined eastern Germany, where there has been a reduction in pollution since the reunification, shows that this reduction has been associated with reductions in the rates of chronic cough and bronchitis symptoms in a new cohort of children [40]. This finding demonstrates not only an association but also the fact that an intervention produces improvements in health.

In the same study location, lung function also improved after the decreases in air pollution in those cities [41]. A further analysis of the Swiss SCARPOL data showed similar results. As particle concentrations fell in Switzerland (from levels well below those in eastern Germany), the prevalence of chronic respiratory symptoms fell in school children. There was considerable variability in how much particle levels fell, which was matched by the rate of improvement in respiratory symptoms.

A similar dramatic effect of intervention was seen in a study by Avol and coworkers [42]. Using the Southern California cohort study mentioned earlier, they identified 110 children who moved from the study area and followed them up in their new home with pulmonary function testing identical to that in the main cohort. Subjects who moved to locations with higher PM_{10} concentrations showed lower rates of annual growth in lung function; subjects who moved to locations with lower PM_{10} concentrations than they had left showed higher rates of growth in lung function. This effect was increased in subjects who lived in the new location for at least 3 years.

Most intriguingly, there is evidence that the mortality associations reported in cohort studies do not represent the effects of lifelong or even long exposures and that mortality rates drop shortly after air pollution levels decline. The first evidence of this finding came from studies looking at natural experiments. Pope and coworkers [43] reported that mortality fell in the Utah Valley in the year a strike closed a steel mill and returned to its previous level the next year, when mill operations resumed. More recently, Clancy and colleagues [44] reported that mortality from heart and lung disease fell in the first winter after a ban on coal sales for domestic heating went into effect in Dublin. There was no evidence that the protective effect increased in subsequent years; it seems to have been realized immediately in the first year.

A new follow-up of the Six City Cohort has examined a further 10 years of mortality experience [45]. In some cities there was a substantial drop in pollution between the first and second follow-up periods, in some cities there was a moderate drop, and in some cities there was little or no change. The mortality rate ratios followed the same pattern: Where there was a substantial drop in pollution there was a substantial improvement in life expectancy; where there was little change in pollution concentrations there was little change in life expectancy.

This pattern fits in well with developing studies that examined shorter term exposure to air pollution, which have extended their gambit to include months. Schwartz [46] examined the association of daily deaths and hospital admissions with air pollution when averaged over different periods after filtering out seasonal and long-term trends [27]. He reported that the size of the air pollution effect increased as one went from days to periods of up to 2 months. At that point, the effect size estimates seemed intermediate between those reported in classical time series and those reported in the cohort studies.

As part of this approach, Schwartz developed a framework for thinking about this question. In this framework, the population is divided into a general pool, with low risk of dying, and a frail pool, with high risk of dying in the near future. Because the causes of frailty can be at least partially reversible (eg, subjects with pneumonia recover, subjects who survive a myocardial infarction have much lower risk of dying in the second month after the infarct than in the first) it is possible to transition back to the general pool from the frail pool, and other events can cause transitions to the frail pool. If the effect of particles on the recruitment rate into, or retention in, the frail pool is greater than the effects of particle exposure on the death rate out of the frail pool, increased exposure will result in an immediate increase in deaths (from the direct effect of particles on the death rate out of the frail pool) and a delayed effect as the increased population of the frail pool results in excess deaths over the next few months.

A frequency domain regression approach by Zeger and coworkers [47] showed similar results. In several studies, Zanobetti and coworkers [48,49] examined the time course of the mortality–death relationship directly using distributed lag models. These models showed a pattern concordant with the hypothesis of Schwartz. There was an immediate increase in deaths after an increase in particle exposure, followed by a long tail of slightly increased deaths that stretched out for 40 days after the initial response. Time series studies by their nature must control for season, which makes it difficult to examine longer lags, but the substantial increase in effect size reported by Zanobetti in these studies suggests that the short- and long-term responses to changes in airborne particles fall on a continuum.

Further support for this theory comes from recent studies that examined pregnancy outcomes and infant mortality. Both responses, by definition, involve exposures of less than a year. For example, Bobak and Leon [50] examined the cross-sectional association between air pollution and infant mortality rates across towns in the Czech Republic. A significant association was seen with particle concentrations. Woodruff and coworkers [51] compared infant death rates in US cities with their levels of PM_{10} in the air. They excluded infant deaths in the first month after birth as likely to reflect complications of pregnancy and delivery and found that PM_{10} was associated with higher death rates in the next 11 months of life. This excess risk seemed to be principally from respiratory illness, although sudden infant death syndrome deaths also were elevated.

Fetal growth and birth weight also have been associated with airborne particles in several studies [52–54]. These data suggest effects of exposures of a year or less. In summary, growing evidence indicates that the relevant averaging time for longer term effects of particulate air pollution may be on the order of a year, rather than decades, and that rapid improvements in health could be expected after reductions in particle exposure.

Summary

Exposure to particles is associated with impairments in respiratory health, including reduced lung function and increased respiratory symptoms. It is also associated with increased risk of dying. The associated reduction in life expectancy is not small, and the strong trend in the risk estimates with improvements in exposure assignment suggests that the actual impact is considerably greater than either the average across studies or the more commonly quoted estimate from the ACS study suggests. Combined with strong evidence from the Six City Study, the Dublin and Utah interventions, and the infant mortality studies suggesting that mortality effects are primarily associated with relatively recent PM exposure and not decade-long exposures, these data suggest a more serious problem and one more amenable to solution than previously thought.

References

[1] Goodhill V. Maimonides: modern medical relevance. Trans Am Acad Ophthalmol Otolaryngol 1971;75(3):463–91.

[2] Chestnut LG, Schwartz J, Savitz DA, et al. Pulmonary function and ambient particulate matter: epidemiological evidence from NHANES I. Arch Environ Health 1991;46(3): 135–44.

[3] Ackermann-Liebrich U, Leuenberger P, Schwartz J, et al. Lung function and long term exposure to air pollutants in Switzerland: Study on Air Pollution and Lung Diseases in Adults (SAPALDIA) team. Am J Respir Crit Care Med 1997;155(1):122–9.

[4] Sekine K, Shima M, Nitta Y, et al. Long term effects of exposure to automobile exhaust on the pulmonary function of female adults in Tokyo, Japan. Occup Environ Med 2004;61(4): 350–7.

[5] Lubinski W, Toczyska I, Chcialowski A, et al. Influence of air pollution on pulmonary function in healthy young men from different regions of Poland. Ann Agric Environ Med 2005; 12(1):1–4.

[6] Schwartz J. Lung function and chronic exposure to air pollution: a cross-sectional analysis of NHANES II. Environ Res 1989;50(2):309–21.

[7] Raizenne M, Neas LM, Damokosh AI, et al. Health effects of acid aerosols on North American children: pulmonary function. Environ Health Perspect 1996;104(5):506–14.

[8] Gauderman WJ, Avol E, Gilliland F, et al. The effect of air pollution on lung development from 10 to 18 years of age. N Engl J Med 2004;351(11):1057–67.

[9] Horak F Jr, Studnicka M, Gartner C, et al. Particulate matter and lung function growth in children: a 3-yr follow-up study in Austrian schoolchildren. Eur Respir J 2002;19(5):838–45.

[10] Dockery DW, Speizer FE, Stram DO, et al. Effects of inhalable particles on respiratory health of children. Am Rev Respir Dis 1989;139(3):587–94.

[11] Braun-Fahrlander C, Vuille JC, Sennhauser FH, et al. Respiratory health and long-term exposure to air pollutants in Swiss schoolchildren. SCARPOL team: Swiss study on childhood allergy and respiratory symptoms with respect to air pollution, climate and pollen. Am J Respir Crit Care Med 1997;155(3):1042–9.

[12] McConnell R, Berhane K, Gilliland F, et al. Air pollution and bronchitic symptoms in Southern California children with asthma. Environ Health Perspect 1999;107(9):757–60.

[13] Dockery DW, Cunningham J, Damokosh AI, et al. Health effects of acid aerosols on North American children: respiratory symptoms. Environ Health Perspect 1996;104(5):500–5.

[14] Lin S, Munsie JP, Hwang SA, et al. Childhood asthma hospitalization and residential exposure to state route traffic. Environ Res 2002;88:73–81.

[15] Gehring U, Cyrys J, Sedlmeir G, et al. Traffic-related air pollution and respiratory health during the first 2 yrs of life. Eur Respir J 2002;19(4):690–8.

[16] Brauer M, Hoek G, Van Vliet P, et al. Air pollution from traffic and the development of respiratory infections and asthmatic and allergic symptoms in children. Am J Respir Crit Care Med 2002;166(8):1092–8.

[17] Venn A, Lewis SA, Cooper M, et al. Living near a main road and the risk of wheezing illness in children. Am J Respir Crit Care Med 2001;164:2177–80.

[18] English P, Neutra R, Scalf R, et al. Examining associations between childhood asthma and traffic flow using a geographic information system. Environ Health Perspect 1999;107(9): 761–7.

[19] Giroux M, Bremont F, Ferrieres J, et al. Exhaled NO in asthmatic children in unpolluted and urban environments. Environ Int 2001;27(4):335–40.

[20] Schwartz J. Particulate air pollution and chronic respiratory disease. Environ Res 1993;62: 7–13.

[21] Abbey DE, Ostro BE, Petersen F, et al. Chronic respiratory symptoms associated with estimated long-term ambient concentrations of fine particulates less than 2.5 microns in aerodynamic diameter (PM2.5) and other air pollutants. J Expo Anal Environ Epidemiol 1995;5: 137–59.

[22] Avino P, De Lisio V, Grassi M, et al. Influence of air pollution on chronic obstructive respiratory diseases: comparison between city (Rome) and hill-country environments and climates. Ann Chim 2004;94:629–34.

[23] Karakatsani A, Andreadaki S, Katsouyanni K, et al. Air pollution in relation to manifestations of chronic pulmonary disease: a nested case-control study in Athens, Greece. Eur J Epidemiol 2003;18:45–53.

[24] Nemery B, Hoet PH, Nemmar A. The Meuse Valley fog of 1930: an air pollution disaster. Lancet 2001;357(9257):704–8.

[25] Her Majesty's Public Health Service Office. Mortality and morbidity during the London Fog of December 1952 [report No 95]. London: Her Majesty's Public Health Service; 1954.

[26] Bell ML, Davis DL. Reassessment of the lethal London fog of 1952: novel indicators of acute and chronic consequences of acute exposure to air pollution. Environ Health Perspect 2001; 109(Suppl 3):389–94.

[27] Schwartz J. Is there harvesting in the association of airborne particles with daily deaths and hospital admissions? Epidemiology 2001;12(1):55–61.

[28] Lave LB, Seskin EP. Air pollution and human health. Science 1970;169(947):723–33.

[29] Chappie M, Lave L. The health effects of air pollution: a reanalysis. J Urban Econ 1982;12: 346–76.

[30] Dockery DW, Pope CA III, Xu X, et al. An association between air pollution and mortality in six US cities. N Engl J Med 1993;329(24):1753–9.

[31] Pope CA III, Thun MJ, Namboodiri MM, et al. Particulate air pollution as a predictor of mortality in a prospective study of US adults. Am J Respir Crit Care Med 1995;151(3 Pt 1):669–74.

[32] Pope CA III, Burnett RT, Thun MJ, et al. Lung cancer, cardiopulmonary mortality, and long-term exposure to fine particulate air pollution. JAMA 2002;287(9):1132–41.

[33] Hoek G, Brunekreef B, Goldbohm S, et al. Association between mortality and indicators of traffic-related air pollution in the Netherlands: a cohort study. Lancet 2002;360(9341): 1203–9.

[34] Willis A, Jerrett M, Burnett RT, et al. The association between sulfate air pollution and mortality at the county scale: an exploration of the impact of scale on a long-term exposure study. J Toxicol Environ Health A 2003;66(16–19):1605–24.

[35] Jerrett M, Burnett RT, Ma R, et al. Spatial analysis of air pollution and mortality in Los Angeles. Epidemiology, 2005;16:727–36.

[36] Filleul L, Rondeau V, Vandentorren S, et al. Twenty five year mortality and air pollution: results from the French PAARC survey. Occup Environ Med 2005;62(7):453–60.

[37] McDonnell WF, Nishino-Ishikawa N, Petersen FF, et al. Relationships of mortality with the fine and coarse fractions of long-term ambient PM10 concentrations in nonsmokers. J Expo Anal Environ Epidemiol 2000;10(5):427–36.

[38] Maheswaran R, Haining RP, Brindley P, et al. Outdoor air pollution and stroke in Sheffield, United Kingdom: a small-area level geographical study. Stroke 2005;36(2):239–43.

[39] Fuchs VR, Frank SR. Air pollution and medical care use by older Americans: a cross-area analysis. Health Aff (Millwood) 2002;21(6):207–14.

[40] Heinrich J, Hoelscher B, Frye C, et al. Improved air quality in reunified Germany and decreases in respiratory symptoms. Epidemiology 2002;13(4):394–401.

[41] Frye C, Hoelscher B, Cyrys J, et al. Association of lung function with declining ambient air pollution. Environ Health Perspect 2003;111(3):383–7.

[42] Avol EL, Gauderman WJ, Tan SM, et al. Respiratory effects of relocating to areas of differing air pollution levels. Am J Respir Crit Care Med 2001;164(11):2067–72.

[43] Pope CA III, Schwartz J, Ransom MR. Daily mortality and PM10 pollution in Utah Valley. Arch Environ Health 1992;47(3):211–7.

[44] Clancy L, Goodman P, Sinclair H, et al. Effect of air-pollution control on death rates in Dublin, Ireland: an intervention study. Lancet 2002;360(9341):1210–4.

[45] Laden F, Schwartz J, Speizer F, et al. Reduction in fine particulate air pollution and mortality: extended follow-up of the Harvard Six Cities Study. Am J Respir Crit Care Med 2006;173:667–72.

[46] Schwartz J. Harvesting and long-term exposure effects in the relationship between air pollution and mortality. Am J Epidemiol 2000;151:440–8.

[47] Zeger SL, Dominici F, Samet J. Harvesting resistant estimates of air pollution effects on mortality. Epidemiology 1999;10:171–5.

[48] Zanobetti A, Wand MP, Schwartz J, et al. Generalized additive distributed lag models: quantifying mortality displacement. Biostatistics 2000;1:279–92.

[49] Zanobetti A, Schwartz J, Samoli E, et al. The temporal pattern of mortality responses to air pollution. Epidemiology 2002;13:87–93.

[50] Bobak M, Leon DA. Air pollution and infant mortality in the Czech Republic, 1986–88. Lancet 1992;340:1010–4.

[51] Woodruff TJ, Grillo J, Schoendorf C. The relationship between selected causes of postneonatal infant mortality and particulate air pollution in the United States. Environ Health Perspect 1997;105:608–12.

[52] Xu X, Ding H, Wang X. Acute effects of total suspended particles and sulfur dioxides on preterm delivery: a community-based cohort study. Arch Environ Health 1995;50:407–15.

[53] Dejmek J, Selevan SG, Benes I, et al. Fetal growth and maternal exposure to particulate matter during pregnancy. Environ Health Perspect 1999;107(6):475–80.

[54] Bobak M, Richards M, Wadsworth M. Air pollution and birth weight in Britain in 1946. Epidemiology 2001;12:358–9.

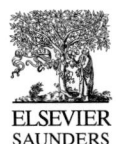

ELSEVIER
SAUNDERS

Clin Occup Environ Med
5 (4) 849–864

CLINICS IN
OCCUPATIONAL AND
ENVIRONMENTAL
MEDICINE

Responses of the Heart to Ambient Particle Inhalation

John J. Godleski, MD

Department of Environmental Health, Harvard School of Public Health,
665 Huntington Avenue, Building II, Room 231, Boston, MA 02115, USA

This article focuses on responses to ambient particles by the heart. Available data from human studies and animal studies are reviewed in an attempt to find a common understanding in the findings. The pathophysiologic mechanisms responsible for these health effects are likely to be complex, and it is highly probable that several different mechanisms work in concert. It is clear that significant cardiovascular morbidity and mortality have been associated with increases in particulate air pollution in epidemiologic time-series studies [1–8]. Changes in blood viscosity [9], decreased heart rate variability [10–17], ST-segment depression [18,19], increased discharges of implanted defibrillators [20,21], increased blood pressure [22–26], and increased circulating markers of inflammation and thrombosis [16,27–30] have been associated with increases in particulate air pollution in various panel and cohort studies.

Laboratory studies also have contributed substantially to understanding the pathophysiologic mechanisms and identifying the components of ambient airborne particles responsible for the adverse effects observed [31,32]. Laboratory advances often have involved studies using ambient particle concentrators that deliver increased concentrations of ambient particle aerosols for inhalation exposure of experimental animals [33–36]. Heart rate variability analysis revealed important disturbances in autonomic tone during exposure of dogs to concentrated ambient particles (CAPs) [37,38]. Although several cardiac outcomes had considerable variability related to day-to-day variability of exposure composition [37,39–41], one of the most consistent responses to CAPs was the increase in the severity of myocardial ischemia during acute coronary artery occlusion in a canine model

This work was supported by grants ES012972 and ES000002 from the National Institutes of Health and Research grant RD83191701 from the US Environmental Protection Agency.

E-mail address: jgodlesk@hsph.harvard.edu

[37,42]. Studies in rodents [43–45], canines [46,47], and people [24,26] suggest that blood vessels may be important targets.

Laboratory studies using ambient particles or surrogates of complex emission sources have suggested inflammatory mechanisms that might plausibly explain effects of particles on the heart [31,32,48,49]. Research has shown that pulmonary inflammation results from inhalation of increased concentrations of ambient particles [27,39–41,50–52], and it has demonstrated that the contribution of combustion-derived components in the composition is important [40,41,43]. Pulmonary inflammation is postulated to be a key intermediary to cardiac effects. The lung may be the source of mediators that cause systemic vascular events. The most compelling evidence to support this concept comes from human studies of military recruits exposed to forest fires in Southeast Asia. These healthy young men had evidence of increases in circulating chemokines or cytokines [51]. Overall, however, the degree of pulmonary inflammation found in most CAPs studies and other inhalation studies using surrogate particles is modest. Inflammatory responses to PM exposure are addressed more fully in the article by Frampton elsewhere in this issue.

Several plausible mechanistic schemes have been proposed to explain the adverse health impact of inhaled ambient particles on the cardiovascular system [2,4]. These schemes include three potential mechanisms for cardiovascular effects of inhaled particles: (1) autonomic nervous system pathways with adverse effects associated with sympathetic nervous system dominance; (2) inflammatory events based on reactive oxygen species generation resulting in some level of lung inflammation with induction of circulating inflammatory and coagulation mediators, which adversely affect the heart and coronary vasculature through endothelial injury, thrombosis, and accelerated atherosclerosis; and (3) direct toxic effects of particulate components on the myocardium or coronary vasculature. Subsequent sections of this article explore data in support of each of these mechanisms and interactions among these mechanisms.

Autonomic nervous system in cardiac responses to inhaled particulate

The autonomic nervous system has been a fruitful focus of investigation. Researchers postulate that particles may trigger neural responses initiated in the respiratory tract [52], and through the autonomic nervous system there can be serious impact on the cardiovascular system [53,54]. Epidemiologic human panel studies [10–17] and laboratory animal studies [37,38] show that changes in heart rate variability occur during exposures to increased levels of ambient particles. These studies suggest an immediate sympathetic response. Heart rate variability is a powerful tool for evaluating autonomic activity because it provides a continuous measure of the interplay between the sympathetic and parasympathetic influences. High-frequency variability provides an indicator of vagal influences, and the low-frequency/

high-frequency ratio provides a measure of the balance between sympathetic and parasympathetic influences. We found important disturbances in heart rate variability, a measure of autonomic function based on the beat-to-beat pattern of heart rate as assessed by spectral analytical methods [37,38]. During CAPs exposure in conscious dogs, autonomic balance is altered in the direction of sympathetic dominance. Human studies also have shown clear associations between increases in particulate air pollution and changes in heart rate variability indicating increases in sympathetic influence [10–15]. Increased propensity to heightened sympathetic tone has been associated with greater risk for arrhythmias and sudden cardiac death [55,56]. In our studies, we also found an increase in the high-frequency component with CAPs exposure, which suggested increased vagal influence [37]. In the presence of endothelial damage, a paradoxical vagal response is observed [57]. The increase in vagal influence also has been seen in some human studies [16]. The role of the vagus nerve and the parasympathetic nervous system in this setting is equally complex. Inhaled irritants usually produce a decrease in heart rate and vasodilatory responses [53]. In our studies with normal animals, it is not surprising that we have found a decrease in heart rate [37,38]. Other researchers have reported similar findings in human and animal studies [53] and increases in heart rate [10–13]. The direction and magnitude of the response may relate to the sympathetic component and either a direct or paradoxical parasympathetic component. It is possible that the vagal response may come about as a compensatory reaction to the increase in sympathetic tone, may be a paradoxical response to endothelial damage, or may be an age-related phenomenon.

The complexity and interrelationships of the autonomic mechanisms are highlighted by a series of recent observations. Using in vivo chemiluminescence, it was found that after CAPs exposure, an increase in lung and cardiac chemiluminescence was detected [58–60]. These measurements represent oxidant activity in the tissues and are used as a measure of oxidative stress. It seemed that increased oxidative activity resulted from the interaction with inhaled particles. This concept was supported in the lung when N-acetylcysteine was used to block the pulmonary response [59]. The cardiac response was more complex, however. Sympathetic and parasympathetic agonists increased cardiac chemiluminescence, and sympathetic and parasympathetic blockers inhibited the response to the agonists and the response to ambient particles using in vivo chemiluminescence [60]. Because sympathetic and parasympathetic agonists significantly increased reactive oxygen species levels and thiobarbituric acid reactive substance accumulation in the heart, it seems that the cardiac chemiluminescence signal may not be caused by the presence of inflammation in the heart, particulate in the heart, or increased cardiac metabolic activity. It is more complex because this observation, which apparently contradicts the basic principle that the sympathetic and parasympathetic systems exert opposite effects on the heart (ie, sympathetic stimulation increases heart rate, whereas parasympathetic stimulation decreases it), may be understood on the basis of the evidence showing that sympathetic and parasympathetic activation can increase the levels of oxidants in cardiac myocytes [61–63]. Consistently, blockade of the receptors of sympathetic and parasympathetic neurotransmitters reduces reactive oxygen species [62], which suggests a receptor-mediated effect on the intracellular sources of reactive oxygen species by sympathetic and parasympathetic transmitters. Chemiluminescence may be a direct measurement of this enhanced sympathetic and parasympathetic influence on the heart and further supports the importance of the role of the autonomic nervous system in the mechanistic response to ambient particles.

Despite large amounts of evidence that inhalation of particles results in autonomic nervous system–mediated cardiac responses, establishing the mechanistic/neurologic pathways and linkages between that inhalation and the resultant autonomic nervous system mediated cardiac outcomes has not been completed. It continues to be an important goal for environmental cardiologic research.

Vascular responses to inhaled particles

The relative sympathetic dominance described previously would be anticipated to increase cardiac contractility, systemic vascular resistance, and, consequently, arterial blood pressure. They all have important ramifications for cardiac health in terms of long-term development of coronary artery disease and hypertensive heart disease. A fundamental measurement of vascular responses to inhaled particulate is systemic blood pressure. Increased blood pressure has been associated with ambient particle exposures [22–26]. Human studies with CAPs and ozone exposure have shown increases in acute arterial vasoconstriction [24] and diastolic blood pressure [64]. A recent study from our laboratory showed statistically significant acute increases in systolic and diastolic blood pressure (each approximately 4 mm Hg) with exposure to CAPs in canines [65]. Unpublished gene expression microarray studies of rat cardiac tissue from our laboratory have shown enormous increases in atrial naturetic peptide, a major mediator of blood pressure reduction in response to blood pressure elevation. Increases in vasoconstriction and blood pressure may be important in the response to ambient particle exposure and could explain several primary cardiac changes, including the finding of ST-segment depression [18,19] with elevated ambient exposure levels and enhanced ischemia with coronary artery occlusion and CAPs exposure [17,20]. Preliminary studies from our laboratory that assessed cardiac perfusion with CAPs or sham exposures showed a decrease in myocardial perfusion with CAPs exposure using the technique of fluorescent microspheres to define perfusion [66–69].

Morphologic changes observed in vessels of the heart from rats exposed to CAPs are illustrated in Fig. 1. These ultrastructural studies are from heart tissue taken for electron microscopy from the same rats whose lungs were

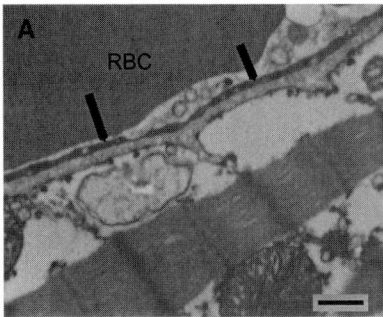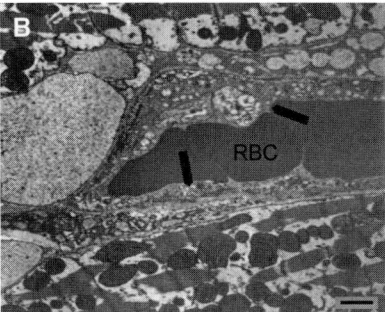

Fig. 1. Ultrastructure of the cardiac vasculature with emphasis on the endothelium of control (sham) exposed rats (*A*) compared with rats exposed to CAPs (*B*). Arrows point to the quiescent endothelium in (*A*) compared with the activated endothelium with CAPs exposure (*B*). In both panels, the red blood cells within the vessel lumens are labeled RBC. (*A*) The entire vessel is not shown, but the endothelium is shown at high magnification. (*B*) More of the vessel is visible, and the endothelium is much thicker, vacuolated, and activated with numerous projections from the endovascular surface. Magnification (*A*) Bar = 0.6 μm; (*B*) Bar = 1.7 μm.

previously reported [40]. The findings include striking endothelial activation and injury in CAPs-exposed animals and lack of these changes in cardiac vasculature of control animals. Such changes may be related to increases in blood pressure, inflammatory endothelial activation, or a combination of these processes. Increases in muscularization and constriction of pulmonary and cardiac vessels have been observed [44,45]. Morphologic studies of the heart and lungs of dogs living in polluted areas of Mexico City compared with dogs from less polluted areas showed marked activation of the endothelium in the dogs from the more polluted area [46,47]. Similar changes in vascular tissue morphology in hypertension and atherosclerotic disease are believed to be associated with changes in levels of mediators that are responsible for controlling the balance of vascular endothelial tone that also may have direct effects on vessel remodeling [70].

Endothelin is a potent mediator of vasoconstriction produced by several lung cells, including endothelial cells, epithelial cells, macrophages, and pulmonary neuroendocrine cells and other tissues [71]. Endothelin-1 is a vasoconstrictor, positive inotrope and chronotrope, and stimulator of the sympathetic nervous system; it has mitogenic properties and stimulates the renin-angiotensin-aldosterone system [71]. Endothelin-1 is chemotactic to monocytes, activates neutrophils, is mitogenic to fibroblasts, has been implicated in creating a hypercoagulable state, and acts as an antifibrinolytic factor [71]. Human studies show that endothelin-1 is increased in response to hypoxemia, heart failure, pulmonary hypertension, asthma, chronic obstructive pulmonary disease, adult respiratory distress syndrome, lung tumors, sepsis, and pulmonary edema [72]. Rats exposed to ambient particles from Ottawa, Canada demonstrated modestly increased plasma levels of endothelin-1 along with histologic changes consistent with lung repair and remodeling [73,74]. Studies in pigs have shown that endothelin-1 produces myocardial ischemia and ventricular arrhythmias via a potent coronary vasoconstrictive effect [71]. Studies show that endothelin increases in human volunteers exposed to CAPs and ozone [24,75]. Gene expression microarray studies from our laboratory also provide evidence of an increase in endothelin gene expression in the lung with CAPs exposure [43].

Nitric oxide (NO) is a short-lived free radical and functions as a potent broncho- and vasodilator, with cytotoxic effects. There are three isoforms of nitric oxide synthetase (NOS), the enzyme that produces NO. They are named for the tissues in which they are found: endothelial cells (eNOS), neurons (nNOS), and, as expressed in macrophages, an inducible isoform (iNOS). NO is expressed by these particular isoforms in many cell types in response to various stimuli; in addition to being a vasodilator, NO also has antiplatelet, antithrombotic, and antimitogenic properties. NO production may in part counterbalance vasoconstrictive responses induced by endothelin production [72]. Studies in our laboratory have shown a substantial decrease in eNOS with CAPs exposure [43]. Our microarray studies after 3 days of CAPs exposure show increases in proinflammatory mediators, increases in vasoconstrictive mediators, and decreases in eNOS [43]. The endothelin/nitric oxide balance is critical in vasomotor control [40–46]. Endothelial injury with decrease in nitric oxide production by the endothelium is recognized as a major mechanism of vasoconstrictive response [71,72]. The balance between NO and endothelins is likely to be a key determinant of acute vasoconstriction resulting from ambient particle exposure.

Although this section has focused on the response of the vessel walls and endothelium, the role of the circulating blood is likely to be important as a transporter of mediators and an active participant via coagulation factors in the responses of vessels. Increased circulating markers of inflammation and thrombosis [16,27–30] have been reported, and important studies have been conducted using diesel and other surrogate particles in studies that define the roles of circulating thrombogenic factors [76–78]. The hypothesis that acute exposure to CAPs causes prothrombotic changes in blood coagulation parameters was examined in a well-controlled study. At multiple time points, six coagulation parameters (platelet count, fibrinogen level, factor VII activity, thrombin-antithrombin complex level, tissue plasminogen activator activity, and plasminogen activator inhibitor activity) were measured, as were all standard blood count parameters. Because there were no consistent exposure-related effects on any of the end points, researchers concluded that this study did not indicate that exposure to CAPs causes adverse effects on blood coagulation in healthy rats [79].

Chronic vascular effects, such as vascular medial wall thickening and the acceleration of atherosclerosis, have been observed in coronary vessels in normal mice [45] and systemic vessels of susceptible models [80,81], all with obvious implications for ischemic heart disease. BALB/c mice were chronically exposed to ambient levels of air pollution in downtown Sao

Paulo, Brazil [45]. The animals were maintained in exposure chambers 24 h/day, 7 days/wk for 4 months. One group was exposed to ambient air, and the control group was exposed to filtered air. Morphometric measurements of the ratio between the lumen and wall areas were performed on transverse sections of renal, pulmonary, and coronary arteries. A significant decrease of lumen/wall ratio with exposure to air pollution was detected in pulmonary ($P = 0.03$) and coronary ($P = 0.021$) arteries, whereas no effects of air pollution were observed in renal vessels [45]. These results indicated that animals chronically exposed to ambient air pollution develop a significant thickening of the arterial wall in the coronary and pulmonary circulation.

In a genetic model of atherosclerotic vascular disease, intratracheal instillation of precollected Ottawa dust caused progression of atherosclerotic lesions toward a more advanced phenotype in Watanabe hyperlipidemic rabbits [80]. Instillation of Ottawa ambient dust also caused an increase in plaque cell turnover and extracellular lipid pools in coronary and aortic lesions and in the total amount of lipids in aortic lesions. These studies showed that progression of atherosclerosis can be related to ambient particulate exposure in a suitable host.

In another study, C57− and ApoE-deficient (ApoE−/−) and ApoE, LDLr (DK)-deficient mice were exposed to concentrated ambient PM2.5 for 6 hours, 5 days/wk for up to 5 months [81]. The overall mean exposure concentration for these groups of animals was 110 μg/m^3. The cross-sectional area of the aortic root of DK mice was examined morphologically using confocal microscopy for the severity of lesion, extent of cellularity, and lipid content. All DK mice—regardless of exposure—had developed extensive lesions in the aortic sinus regions, with lesion areas that covered more than 79% of the total area. In male DK mice, the lesion areas in the aortic sinus regions seemed to be enhanced by CAPs, with changes approaching statistical significance. Plaque cellularity was increased significantly (28%), whereas there were no CAPs-associated changes in the lipid content in these mice. When examining the entire aorta opened longitudinally, the ApoE−/− and DK mice had prominent areas of severe atherosclerosis covering 40% or more of the lumenal surface. Visual examination suggested that plaques tend to form in clusters concentrating near the aortic arch and the iliac bifurcations. Quantitative measurements showed that CAPs exposure significantly increased the percentage of aortic intimal surface covered by grossly discernible atherosclerotic lesion by 57% in the ApoE−/− mice [81]. In this study, subchronic CAPs exposure in mice prone to develop atherosclerotic lesions had a significant impact on the size, severity, and composition of aortic atherosclerotic plaques.

Acute and chronic effects of inhaled particles on the systemic vasculature and the coronary vascular system have been demonstrated. It remains to be determined whether the changes observed are secondary to the elevation of blood pressure or caused by a more direct effect of the particles. Although currently more direct evidence seems to support the possibility that the vascular changes observed may be more related to the effect of blood pressure changes, it is likely that both mechanisms play a role. Ongoing studies will find more evidence of direct vascular effects.

Myocardial ischemia with inhalation of ambient particles

Long-term follow-up of the American Cancer Society cohort has provided a large database to assess the effect of chronic exposure to various levels of air pollution and relate increased levels of particulate pollution to specific causes of death [1,8,26]. In a recent study, exposure to increased levels of particles were most strongly associated with mortality attributable to ischemic heart disease, dysrhythmias, heart failure, and cardiac arrest [26]. For these cardiovascular causes of death, a 10-$\mu g/m^3$ elevation in fine particulate matter was associated with 8% to 18% increases in mortality risk, with comparable or larger risks being observed for smokers relative to nonsmokers. When the data were stratified by smoking status, the most dramatic increase in relative risk was found in smokers with hypertension, which suggested a synergistic response in particulate matter-related mortality between smoking and hypertension [26]. This study solidified the importance of ischemic heart disease and hypertension as important disease processes related to chronically elevated ambient particulate pollution.

The relationship of the acute onset of myocardial infarction to ambient particulate pollution has been the subject of several studies [54,82]. In one study [82], a highly significant association ($P < 0.001$) was found between exposure to traffic and the onset of a myocardial infarction within 1 hour afterward. The time the subjects spent in cars, on public transportation, or on motorcycles or bicycles was consistently linked with an increase in the risk of myocardial infarction. To link inflammatory mechanisms with autonomic responses, an underlying supposition is that important factors such as cytokines, which are generated as part of the inflammatory response to ambient particulate, could affect autonomic tone through pulmonary reflexes and direct action on the central nervous system. Our studies with a canine coronary occlusion model show that there are immediate and persistent effects of ambient particulate on enhanced ischemia [37,42]. When the onset of myocardial infarction was associated with ambient air pollution in epidemiologic studies, significant relationships to ambient particles were found on the day of infarction [54,82] and the previous day [54], which indicates that there is an immediate and protracted effect of particulate pollution in people. The similarity between the human and canine studies is remarkable. Regardless of whether the immediate effect is mediated via the autonomic nervous system or whether the protracted component is caused by an inflammatory response, the impact seems to be on the coronary vasculature in both instances.

In canine studies, CAPs exposure shortens the time to develop an elevation of the ST-segment and increases peak ST-segment levels during a 5-minute period of total left anterior descending coronary artery occlusion in chronically instrumented dogs [37,42]. These observations suggest heightened risk for increased infarct size and arrhythmias during acute vessel obstruction. Human studies that demonstrate associations between increases in ambient particulate and the onset of myocardial infarction underscore the relevance and importance of these findings [54,82]. If these studies are interpreted in relationship to the vascular findings described previously, it seems that the morphologic endothelial changes of the small vasculature of the heart coupled with or resulting in a decrease in coronary vascular perfusion associated with CAPs exposure are likely to explain these findings. Understanding the relationships among coronary artery blood flow, systemic vascular resistance, and changes in myocardial work resulting from inhalation of particles is critical in understanding changes in ischemia that results from particle inhalation. The implication of increased infarct size with particle exposure is an important observation that must be studied in human populations and with further confirmation in animals. Such animal studies are underway in our laboratory using fluorescent microsphere techniques to assess myocardial perfusion with the coronary occlusion model and CAPs or sham exposures [66–69]. Although this question might be difficult to approach in human studies, retrospective studies using clinical imaging techniques, electrocardiogram analyses, and clinical laboratory levels of troponin or other injury markers might be able to relate a measure of extent of myocardial infarction to ambient air pollution levels.

Another remarkable similarity between recent human studies [82] and our canine studies [42] is the source of ambient particles responsible for the findings. The human studies clearly relate the onset on myocardial infarction to traffic. In our studies, the increased elevation of the S-T segment is most significantly related to silicon as a tracer in univariate and multivariate analyses. In our urban setting, this tracer is considered a marker for urban road dust and all its constituents. The human and animal studies relate myocardial ischemic effects to traffic factors.

Because epidemiologic studies show an increase in implanted defibrillator discharge with increases in ambient particulate [20,21], a model system to study the role of ambient particle pollution on the generation of cardiac arrhythmias is needed. Because the period immediately after an acute myocardial infarction is recognized as a highly vulnerable period for the development of fatal arrhythmias, animal studies have been conducted to assess whether inhaled particle exposure can increase arrhythmias during this vulnerable stage of acute myocardial infarction [83,84]. Marked increases in post–myocardial infarction arrhythmia were found in rats exposed by inhalation to aerosols of residual oil fly ash [83]. The effect of exposure to CAPs and gaseous traffic related pollutants, such as carbon monoxide (CO), have been assessed on arrhythmia incidence [84]. CO exposure reduced ventricular premature beat frequency by 60.4% ($P = 0.012$) during the exposure period compared with controls. This effect was modified by infarct type and the number of pre-exposure ventricular premature beats and was not mediated through changes in heart rate. CAPs exposure increased ventricular premature beat frequency during the exposure period. This effect was modified by the number of pre-exposure ventricular premature beats. Overall, neither CAPs nor CO had any effect on heart rate, but CAPs increased heart rate in specific subgroups. No significant interactions were observed between the effects of CO at high ambient concentration levels and CAPs. In this animal model, the responses to CO and CAPs are distinctly different. Studies of particle exposures immediately after acute myocardial infarction in rats can serve as a model to assess the development of cardiac arrhythmias caused by inhalation of ambient particulate and to assess directly the individual roles of important co-pollutants, such as CO and ambient particulate, whose effects are difficult to disentangle in human studies.

Direct effects of ambient particulate on the heart

The question of whether inhaled particles can translocate to the heart to have a direct effect on myocardial contraction, conduction, repolarization, or arrhythmia development has not yet been answered. Nor has the possibility of a direct effect on the vascular endothelium been demonstrated conclusively. It is clear, however, that some ultrafine particles and nanoparticles can cross the pulmonary epithelium [85–87] and have a systemic distribution [88–90], and the distribution pattern seems to be related to the composition of the particles [91,92]. Identification of environmental particles in cardiac macrophages of rats has been reported [34,46]. The elemental signatures by analytical electron microscopy of particles found in cardiac macrophages from an aerosol fly ash exposure are illustrated in Fig. 2. In this study, the cardiac macrophages had immunohistochemical evidence of induction of the proinflammatory cytokine MIP-2 in their cytoplasm [93]. Conclusive proof of the association of translocated particles to the local induction of cytokines in the heart is lacking, however. A recent study using ultrafine carbon particles in WKY rats assessed several outcomes, including those that might indicate a direct effect on the heart [94]. Evidence was found for autonomic nervous system effects on the heart (eg, increased heart rate and decreased heart rate variability), but no evidence was found of effects on coagulation parameters, inflammation as a mechanism of cardiac effects, or direct effects on the heart.

Whether particles redistribute systemically as particles or whether dissolution of inhaled particulate takes place in the lung and redistribution takes place of the dissolved form seems to be an argument of little consequence. The most important issue is whether systemic redistributions of toxic constituents in biologically active or potentially active forms take place. Developing information to understand fully the health effects and consequence of

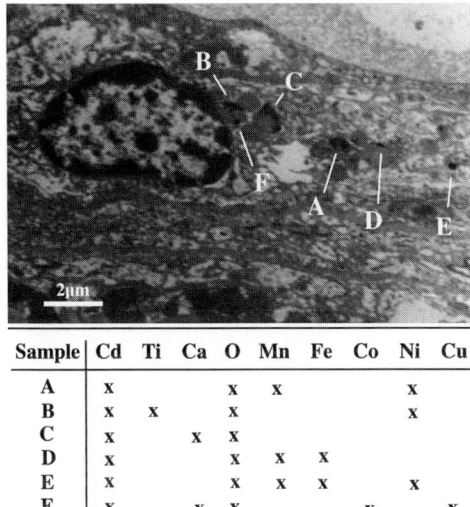

Sample	Cd	Ti	Ca	O	Mn	Fe	Co	Ni	Cu
A	x			x	x			x	
B	x	x		x				x	
C	x		x	x					
D	x			x	x	x			
E	x			x	x	x		x	
F	x		x	x			x		x

Fig. 2. A rat cardiac macrophage from an animal exposed to an oil fly ash aerosol is illustrated. The macrophage contains six groups of ultrafine particles labeled A to F. The elemental composition of the particle groups determined by electron energy loss spectroscopy and spectroscopic imaging includes several metallic elements as oxides, most notably nickel, cadmium, and manganese. Iron, calcium copper, titanium, and cobalt are also present. Magnification: Bar = 2 μm.

such redistributions should be a high priority in this field of research. In a study considered a classic in cardiac toxicology published in 1971, Rheinhardt and colleagues [95] showed that organic vapor aerosols resulted in cardiac arrhythmias. Studies have shown that organic materials, such as particulate benzo(a)pyrene, which rapidly leave the lung, are found in the circulation within seconds of inhalation and can undergo biotransformation and continue to circulate [96,97]. Benzo(a)pyrene also has been shown to have dramatic effects on vascular smooth muscle cells in culture [98,99] Although not specifically shown to have effects on the myocardium, it is clearly possible that the changes in vascular cells seen in vitro could account for many of the pathophysiologic in vivo changes observed with cardiac vessels.

Soluble metal ions and other agents at relatively high concentrations in vitro have been studied with cultured cardiac myocytes and have been shown to have effects on conduction and repolarization [100]. These studies must be revisited in relationship to levels of materials that could be released in vivo with ambient particulate pollution. Common mechanisms applicable to toxic organic species, metals, and other potential toxicants in ambient particles must be considered in understanding final common pathways of direct effects on coronary vessels, cardiac myocytes, and specialized cells of cardiac electrical signal conduction. A leading candidate for a common mechanism is the generation of reactive oxygen species, which is known to occur with cellular interactions of metals and organics [98,101]. Reactive oxygen species also may be generated through autonomic nervous system stimulation and ischemia reperfusion mechanisms [101]. Although the possibility of demonstrating that a single mechanism might explain all phenomena relating to responses of the heart to ambient particles is attractive, the current state of understanding and proof is far from this point.

References

[1] Pope CA III. Epidemiological evidence of relationship between particle exposure and cardiovascular outcomes. In: Heinrich U, Mohr U, editors. Relationships between acute and chronic effects of air pollution. Washington, DC: ILSI Press; 2000. p. 115–28.

[2] Brook RD, Franklin B, Cascio W, et al. Air pollution and cardiovascular disease: a statement for healthcare professionals from the expert panel on population and prevention science of the American Heart Association. Circulation 2004;109:2655–71.

[3] Barclay J, Hillis G, Ayres J. Air pollution and the heart: cardiovascular effects and mechanisms. Toxicol Rev 2005;24:115–23.

[4] Delfino RJ, Sioutas C, Malik S. Potential role of ultrafine particles in associations between airborne particle mass and cardiovascular health. Environ Health Perspect 2005;113: 934–46.

[5] Schwartz J, Morris R. Air pollution and hospital admissions for cardiovascular disease in Detroit, Michigan. Am J Epidemiol 1995;142:23–35.

[6] Schwartz J. Air pollution and hospital admissions for heart disease in eight US counties. Epidemiology 1999;10:17–22.

[7] Burnett RT, Dales R, Krewski D, et al. Associations between ambient particulate sulfate and admissions to Ontario hospitals for cardiac and respiratory diseases. Am J Epidemiol 1995;142:15–22.

[8] Pope CA III, Burnett RT, Thun MJ, et al. Lung cancer, cardiopulmonary mortality, and long-term exposure to fine particulate air pollution. JAMA 2002;287:1132–41.

[9] Peters A, Doring A, Wichmann HE, et al. Increased plasma viscosity during the 1985 air pollution episode: a link to mortality? Lancet 1997;349:1582–7.

[10] Liao D, Creason J, Shy C, et al. Daily variation of particulate air pollution and poor cardiac autonomic control in the elderly. Environ Health Perspect 1999;107:521–5.

[11] Pope CA III, Verrier RL, Lovett EG, et al. Heart rate variability associated with particulate air pollution. Am Heart J 1999;138(5 Pt 1):890–9.

[12] Gold DR, Litonjua A, Schwartz J, et al. Ambient pollution and heart rate variability. Circulation 2000;101(11):1267–73.

[13] Magari SR, Hauser R, Schwartz J, et al. Association of heart rate variability with occupational and environmental exposure to particulate air pollution. Circulation 2001;104: 986–91.

[14] Devlin RB, Ghio AJ, Kehrl H, et al. Elderly humans exposed to concentrated air pollution particles have decreased heart rate variability. Eur Respir J 2003;(Suppl 40):76S–80S.

[15] Park SK, O'Neill MS, Vokonas PS, et al. Effects of air pollution on heart rate variability: the VA Normative Aging Study. Environ Health Perspect 2005;113:304–9.

[16] Riediker M, Cascio WE, Griggs TR, et al. Particulate matter exposure in cars is associated with cardiovascular effects in healthy young men. Am J Respir Crit Care Med 2004;169: 934–40.

[17] Vallejo M, Ruiz S, Hermosillo AG, et al. Ambient fine particles modify heart rate variability in young healthy adults. J Expo Anal Environ Epidemiol 2006;16:125–30.

[18] Pekkanen J, Peters A, Hoek G, et al. Particulate air pollution and risk of ST segment depression during repeated submaximal exercise tests among subjects with coronary heart disease: the ULTRA study. Circulation 2002;106(8):933–8.

[19] Gold DR, Litonjua AA, Zanobetti A, et al. Air pollution and ST-segment depression in elderly subjects. Environ Health Perspect 2005;113:883–7.

[20] Peters A, Liu E, Verrier RL, et al. Air pollution and incidence of cardiac arrhythmia. Epidemiology 2000;11:11–7.

[21] Dockery DW, Luttmann-Gibson H, Rich DO, et al. Association of air pollution with increased incidence of ventricular tachyarrhythmias recorded by implanted cardioverter defibrillators. Environ Health Perspect 2005;113:670–4.

[22] Linn WS, Gong H Jr, Clark KW, et al. Day-to-day particulate exposures and health changes in Los Angeles area residents with severe lung disease. J Air Waste Manag Assoc 1999;49:108–15.

[23] Ibald-Mulli A, Stieber J, Wichmann HE, et al. Effects of air pollution on blood pressure: a population based approach. Am J Public Health 2001;91:571–7.

[24] Brook RD, Brook JR, Urch B, et al. Inhalation of fine particulate air pollution and ozone causes acute arterial vasoconstriction in healthy adults. Circulation 2002;105:1534–6.

[25] Zanobetti A, Canner MJ, Stone PH, et al. Ambient pollution and blood pressure in cardiac rehabilitation patients. Circulation 2004;110:2184–9.

[26] Pope CA, Burnett RT, Thurston GD, et al. Cardiovascular mortality and long-term exposure to particulate air pollution: epidemiological evidence of general pathophysiological pathways of disease. Circulation 2004;109:71–7.

[27] Ghio AJ, Kim C, Devlin RB. Concentrated ambient air particles induce mild pulmonary inflammation in healthy human volunteers. Am J Respir Crit Care Med 2000;162:981–8.

[28] Schwartz J. Air pollution and blood markers of cardiovascular risk. Environ Health Perspect 2001;109(Suppl 3):405–9.

[29] Pope CA, Hansen ML, Long RW, et al. Ambient particulate air pollution, heart rate variability, and blood markers of inflammation in a panel of elderly subjects. Environ Health Perspect 2004;112:339–45.

[30] Ruckerl R, Ibald-Mulli A, Koenig W, et al. Air pollution and markers of inflammation and coagulation in patients with coronary heart disease. Am J Respir Crit Care Med 2006;173:432–41.

[31] Costa DL. Particulate matter and cardiopulmonary health: a perspective. Inhal Toxicol 2000;12(Suppl 3):35–44.

[32] Ghio AJ, Huang YC. Exposure to concentrated ambient particles (CAPs): a review. Inhal Toxicol 2004;16:53–9.

[33] Sioutas C, Koutrakis P, Godleski JJ, et al. Fine particle concentrators for inhalation exposures: effect of particle size and composition. J Aerosol Sci 1997;28:1057–71.

[34] Godleski JJ, Clarke RE. Systemic responses to inhaled ambient particles: pathophysiologic mechanisms of cardiopulmonary effects. In: Heyder J, Gehr P, editors. Particle-lung interactions: lung biology in health and disease series. New York: Marcel Dekker; 2000. p. 577–601.

[35] Lawrence J, Koutrakis P, Godleski J. Performance stability of the Harvard ambient particles concentrator. Aerosol Sci Technol 2004;38:219–27.

[36] Savage ST, Lawrence J, Katz T, et al. Does the Harvard/Environmental Protection Agency ambient particle concentrator change the toxic potential of particles? J Air Waste Manage Assoc 2003;53:1088–97.

[37] Godleski JJ, Verrier RL, Koutrakis P, et al. Mechanisms of morbidity and mortality from exposure to ambient air particles. Health Effects Institute Research Report 2000;91:1–103.

[38] Godleski JJ. Cardiovascular responses to inhaled particles. In: Heinrich U, Mohr U, editors. Relationships between acute and chronic effects of air pollution. Washington, DC: ILSI Press; 2000. p. 141–55.

[39] Kodavanti UP, Mebane R, Ledbetter A, et al. Variable pulmonary responses from exposure to concentrated ambient air particles in rat model of bronchitis. Toxicol Sci 2000;54: 441–51.

[40] Saldiva PHN, Clarke RW, Coull BA, et al. Acute pulmonary inflammation induced by concentrated ambient air particles is related to particle composition. Am J Respir Crit Care Med 2002;165:1610–7.

[41] Clarke RW, Coull B, Reinisch U, et al. Inhaled concentrated ambient particles are associated with hematologic and bronchoalveolar lavage changes in canines. Environ Health Perspect 2000;108(12):1179–87.

[42] Wellenius GA, Coull BA, Godleski JJ, et al. Inhalation of concentrated ambient air particles exacerbates myocardial ischemia in conscious dogs. Environ Health Perspect 2003;111:402–8.

[43] Godleski JJ, Clarke RW, Coull BA, et al. Composition of inhaled urban air particles determines acute pulmonary responses. Ann Occup Hyg 2002;46(Suppl 1):419–24.

[44] Batalha JRF, Saldiva PHN, Clarke RW, et al. Concentrated ambient air particles induce vasoconstriction of small pulmonary arteries in rats. Environ Health Perspect 2002;110: 1191–7.

[45] Lemos M, Mohallem S, Macchione M, et al. Chronic exposure to urban air pollution induces structural alterations in murine coronary arteries. Inhal Tox 2006;18: 247–53.

[46] Calderon-Garciduenas L, Gambling TM, Acuna H, et al. Canines as sentinel species for assessing chronic exposures to air pollutants: II. Cardiac pathology. Toxicol Sci 2001;61(2): 356–67.

[47] Calderon-Garciduenas L, Mora-Tiscareno A, Fordham LA, et al. Canines as sentinel species for assessing chronic exposures to air pollutants: I. Respiratory pathology. Toxicol Sci 2001;61(2):342–55.

[48] Donaldson K, Stone V, Seaton A, et al. Ambient particle inhalation and the cardiovascular system: potential mechanisms. Environ Health Perspect 2001;109(Suppl 4):523–7.

[49] Utell MJ, Frampton MW, Zareba W, et al. Cardiovascular effects associated with air pollution: potential mechanisms and methods of testing. Inhal Toxicol 2002;14(12): 1231–47.

[50] Clarke RW, Catalano PJ, Koutrakis P, et al. Urban air particulate inhalation alters pulmonary function and induces pulmonary inflammation in a rodent model of chronic bronchitis. Inhal Toxicol 1999;11:637–56.

[51] van Eeden S, Tan W, Suwa T, et al. Cytokines involved in the systemic inflammatory response induced by exposure to particulate matter air pollutants (PM(10)). Am J Respir Crit Care Med 2001;164(5):826–30.

[52] Carr M, Undern B. Inflammation-induced plasticity of the afferent innervation of the airways. Environ Health Perspect 2001;109(Suppl 4):567–71.

[53] Widdicombe J, Lee L. Airway reflexes, autonomic function, and cardiovascular responses. Environ Health Perspect 2001;109(Suppl 4):579–84.

[54] Peters A, Dockery DW, Muller JE, et al. Increased particulate air pollution and the triggering of myocardial infarction. Circulation 2001;103(23):2810–5.

[55] Kleiger R, Miller JP, Bigger JT Jr, et al. Decreased heart rate variability and its association with increased mortality after acute myocardial infarction. Am J Cardiol Clin 1987;59: 256–62.

[56] Bigger JJ, Fleiss JL, Steinman RC, et al. Frequency domain measures of heart period variability and mortality after myocardial infarction. Circulation 1992;85:164–71.

[57] Ludmer P, Selwyn AP, Shook TL, et al. Paradoxical vasoconstriction induced by acetylcholine in atherosclerotic coronary arteries. N Engl J Med 1986;294:1045–51.

[58] Gurgueira SA, Lawrence J, Coull B, et al. Rapid increases in the steady-state concentration of reactive oxygen species in the lungs and heart after particulate air pollution inhalation. Environ Health Perspect 2002;110(8):749–55.

[59] Rhoden CR, Lawrence J, Godleski JJ, et al. N-acetylcysteine prevents lung inflammation after short-term inhalation exposure to concentrated ambient particles. Toxicol Sci 2004; 79(2):296–303.

[60] Rhoden CR, Wellenius G, Ghelfi E, et al. PM-induced cardiac oxidative stress is mediated by autonomic stimulation. Biochim Biophys Acta 2005;1725:305–13.

[61] Cohen MV, Yang XM, Liu GS, et al. Acetylcholine, bradykinin, opioids, and phenylephrine, but not adenosine, trigger preconditioning by generating free radicals and opening mitochondrial K(ATP) channels. Circ Res 2001;89:273–8.

[62] Krieg T, Philipp S, Cui L, et al. Peptide blockers of PKG inhibit ROS generation by acetylcholine and bradykinin in cardiomyocytes but fail to block protection in the whole heart. Am J Physiol Heart Circ Physiol 2005;288:H1976–81.

[63] Krieg T, Qin Q, Philipp S, et al. Acetylcholine and bradykinin trigger preconditioning in the heart through a pathway that includes Akt and NOS. Am J Physiol Heart Circ Physiol 2004;287:H2606–11.

[64] Urch B, Silverman F, Corey P, et al. Acute blood pressure responses in healthy adults during controlled air pollution exposures. Environ Health Perspect 2005;113:1052–5.

[65] Bartoli CR, Diaz EA, Lawrence J, et al. Exposure to concentrated ambient air particles raises systemic blood pressure in canines [abstract]. Proc Am Thorac Soc 2006;3:A551.

[66] Bassingthwaighte J, Malone MA, Moffett TC, et al. Molecular and particulate depositions for regional myocardial flows in sheep. Circ Res 1990;66:1328–44.

[67] Abel F, Cooper RH, Beck RR. Use of fluorescent latex microspheres to measure coronary blood flow distribution. Circ Shock 1993;41:156–61.

[68] Chien G, Anselone CG, Davis RF, et al. Fluorescent vs. radioactive microsphere measurement of regional myocardial blood flow. Cardiovasc Res 1995;30:405–12.

[69] Glenny R, Bernard S, Brinkley M. Validation of fluorescent-labeled microspheres for measurement of regional organ perfusion. J Appl Physiol 1993;74:2585–97.

[70] Gray G. Generation of endothelin. In: Gray G, Webb DJ, editors. Molecular biology and pharmacology of the endothelins. Austin (TX): Landes Bioscience; 1995. p. 13–32.

[71] Gianessi D, Del Ry S, Vitale RL, et al. The role of endothelins and their receptors in heart failure. Pharm Res 2001;43(2):11–126.

[72] Chen Y, Oparil S. Endothelial dysfunction in the pulmonary vascular bed. Am J Med Sci 2000;320(4):223–32.

[73] Vincent R, Kumarathasan P, Goegan P, et al. Inhalation toxicology of urban ambient particulate matter: acute cardiovascular effects in rats. Cambridge (MA): Health Effects Institute; 2001. p. 5–54.

[74] Bouthillier L, Vincent R, Goegan P, et al. Acute effects of inhaled urban particles and ozone: lung morphology, macrophage activity, and plasma endothelin-1. Am J Pathol 1998;153:1873–84.

[75] Vincent R, Kumarathasan P, Mukherjee B, et al. Exposure to urban particles (pm 2.5) causes elevations of the plasma vasopeptides endothelin (ET)-1 and ET-3 in humans. Am J Respir Crit Care Med 2001;163:A313.

[76] Nemmar A, Hoet PH, Dinsdale D, et al. Diesel exhaust particles in lung acutely enhance experimental peripheral thrombosis. Circulation 2003;107(8):1202–8.

[77] Nemmar A, Hoet PH, Vanquickenborne B, et al. Passage of inhaled particles into the blood circulation in humans. Circulation 2002;105(4):411–4.

[78] Frampton MW. Systemic and cardiovascular effects of airway injury and inflammation: ultrafine particle exposure in humans. Environ Health Perspect 2001;109(Suppl 4): 529–32.

[79] Nadziejko C, Fang K, Chen LC, et al. Effect of concentrated ambient particulate matter on blood coagulation parameters in rats. Res Rep Health Eff Inst 2002;111:7–29 [discussion: 31–8].

[80] Suwa T, Hogg JC, Quinlan KB, et al. Particulate air pollution induces progression of atherosclerosis. Am Coll Cardiol 2002;39:935–42.

[81] Chen LC, Nadziejko C. Effects of subchronic exposures to concentrated ambient particles (CAPs) in mice: VCAPs exacerbate aortic plaque development in hyperlipidemic mice. Inhal Toxicol 2005;17:217–24.

[82] Peters A, von Klot S, Heier M, et al. Exposure to traffic and the onset of myocardial infarction. N Engl J Med 2004;351:1721–30.

[83] Wellenius G, Saldiva PHN, Batalha JR, et al. Exposure to residual oil fly ash (ROFA) particles exacerbates the effects of myocardial infarction in rat. Toxicol Sci 2002;66:327–35.

[84] Wellenius GA, Batalha JRF, Diaz EA, et al. Cardiac effects of carbon monoxide and ambient particles in a rat model of myocardial infarction. Toxicol Sci 2004;80:367–76.

[85] Stearns RC, Paulauskis JD, Godleski JJ. Endocytosis of ultrafine particles by A549 cells. Am J Respir Cell Mol Biol 2001;24:108–15.

[86] Kapp N, Kreyling W, Schulz H, et al. Electron energy loss spectroscopy for analysis of inhaled ultrafine particles in rat lungs. Microsc Res Tech 2004;63:298–305.

[87] Geiser M, Rothen-Rutishauser B, Kapp N, et al. Ultrafine particles cross cellular membranes by nonphagocytic mechanisms in lungs and in cultured cells. Environ Health Perspect 2005;113:1555–60.

[88] Nemmar A, Vanbilloen H, Hoylaerts MF, et al. Passage of intratracheally instilled ultrafine particles from the lung into the systemic circulation in hamster. Am J Respir Crit Care Med 2001;164:1665–8.

[89] Oberdörster G, Sharp Z, Atudorei V, et al. Extrapulmonary translocation of ultrafine carbon particles following whole-body inhalation exposure of rats. J Toxicol Environ Health 2002;65:1531–43.

[90] Brown JS, Zeman KL, Bennett WD. Ultrafine particle deposition and clearance in the healthy and obstructed lung. Am J Respir Crit Care Med 2002;166:1240–7.

[91] Kreyling WG, Semmler M, Erbe F, et al. Translocation of ultrafine insoluble iridium particles from lung epithelium to extrapulmonary organs is size dependent but very low. J Toxicol Environ Health 2002;65:1513–30.

[92] Oberdörster G, Sharp Z, Atudorei V, et al. Translocation of inhaled ultrafine particles to the brain. Inhal Toxicol 2004;16:437–45.

[93] Killingsworth C, Alessandrini F, Krishna Murthy G, et al. Inflammation chemokine expression and death in monocrotaline-treated rats following fuel oil fly ash inhalation. Inhal Toxicol 1997;9:541–65.

[94] Harder V, Gilmour P, Lentner B, et al. Cardiovascular responses in unrestrained WKY rats to inhaled ultrafine carbon particles. Inhal Toxicol 2005;17:29–42.

[95] Reinhardt C, Azar A, Maxfield M, et al. Cardiac arrhythmias and aerosol sniffing. Arch Environ Health 1971;22:265–79.

[96] Gerde P, Muggenburg BA, Lundborg M, et al. The rapid alveolar absorption of diesel soot-adsorbed benzo[a]pyrene: bioavailability, metabolism and dosimetry of an inhaled particle-borne carcinogen. Carcinogenesis 2001;22:741–9.

[97] Ramesh A, Greenwood M, Inyang F, et al. Toxicokinetics of inhaled benzo[a]pyrene: plasma and lung bioavailability. Inhal Toxicol 2001;13:533–53.

[98] Ramos KS. Redox regulation of c-Ha-ras and osteopontin signaling in vascular smooth muscle cells: implications in chemical atherogenesis. Annu Rev Pharmacol Toxicol 1999; 29:243–65.

[99] Johnson CD, Balagurunathan Y, Lu KP, et al. Genomic profiles and predictive biological networks in oxidant-induced atherogenesis. Physiol Genomics 2003;13:263–75.

[100] Melchert RB, Joseph J, Kennedy RH. Interaction of xenobiotics with myocardial signal transduction pathways. Cardiovasc Toxicol 2002;2:1–23.

[101] Nel A. Air pollution-related illness: effects of particles. Science 2005;308:804–6.

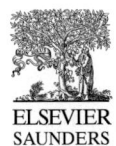

ELSEVIER
SAUNDERS

Clin Occup Environ Med
5 (4) 865–881

CLINICS IN
OCCUPATIONAL AND
ENVIRONMENTAL
MEDICINE

Effects of Particulate Air Pollution on Hemostasis

Abderrahim Nemmar, DVM, PhD[a,c],
Marc F. Hoylaerts, PhD[b],
Benoit Nemery, MD, PhD[a],*

[a]K.U. Leuven, Laboratory of Pneumology (Unit of Lung Toxicology), Herestraat 49,
B-3000, Leuven, Belgium
[b]K.U. Leuven, Center for Molecular and Vascular Biology, Herestraat 49, B-3000,
Leuven, Belgium
[c]Department of Physiology, Sultan Qaboos University, College of Medicine, P.O. Box 35,
Al-khod 123, Sultanate of Oman

Urban air pollution consists of a complex mixture of gaseous and particulate agents. Most published studies concur with the statement that although gaseous pollutants, such as ozone or SO_2, play a significant role, the unifying element of the adverse health effects of urban air pollution consists of respirable particles [1–3]. During the past decade, a large body of epidemiologic studies linking particulate air pollution and increased cardiovascular morbidity and mortality has been reported [4]. Several studies have shown that associations between particulate matter (PM) with a diameter equal or lower than 10 μm (PM_{10}) and mortality persist even at low concentrations of air pollutants [1,5,6]. These epidemiologic observations have demonstrated that peaks of air pollution not only have respiratory effects but also increase cardiovascular morbidity and mortality [7]. More people die from cardiovascular than from pulmonary diseases during episodes of urban air pollution [8]. A growing number of epidemiologic and clinical studies support the concept that components of the cardiovascular system are affected by particulate air pollutants [9,10]. PM has been associated with increased plasma viscosity [11], changes in blood parameters (eg, fibrinogen levels or red blood cell counts) [12], arterial vasoconstriction [13], increased heart rate [14], elevated systolic blood pressure [15], and decreased heart rate variability [10]. These effects can be responsible for pathophysiologic changes in cardiac function,

---

* Corresponding author.
  E-mail address: ben.nemery@med.kuleuven.ac.be (B. Nemery).

1526-0046/06/$ - see front matter © 2006 Elsevier Inc. All rights reserved.
doi:10.1016/j.coem.2006.07.007

such as reported in PM-related exacerbations in patients with ischemic heart disease [16], cardiac arrhythmias [17], and congestive heart failure [18]. Peters and colleagues [19], using a case-crossover approach, interviewed 772 patients with acute myocardial infarction and found that elevated concentrations of $PM_{2.5}$ (PM with a diameter <2.5 μm) were associated with a transient risk of acute myocardial infarction onset during two separate time windows (ie, within 2 hours and 1 day after exposure). More recently, the same authors assessed the association between onset of a nonfatal myocardial infarction and exposure to traffic [20]. They observed an association between exposure to traffic while traveling in cars, buses, and trolley cars and while riding on a bicycle or motorcycle and the onset of a myocardial infarction within 1 hour afterward.

Künzli and colleagues [21] studied the association between long-term exposure to $PM_{2.5}$ and carotid intima-media thickness in subjects living in different areas of Los Angeles. Subjects who lived in the areas with highest annual mean concentrations of ambient $PM_{2.5}$ had greater increases in intima-media thickness.

Although the body of evidence suggests that the relationship between PM and cardiovascular morbidity and mortality is causal, the mechanisms behind these associations are not fully understood [7]. To confer biologic plausibility for these consistent epidemiologic observations, several research groups have begun investigating the possible mechanisms linking inhaled PM and cardiovascular endpoints [22]. Currently, three lines of particle-related research are being pursued [7,22–24]. According to one research line, inhaled particles are suggested to impact on the autonomic nervous system and lead to changes in the pattern of breathing, heart rate, and heart rate variability. A second line has explored whether and how inhaled particles affect the cardiovascular system through inflammatory mediators produced in the lungs and released into the circulation. A third line of research focuses on the possibility that ultrafine particles (UFPs) with a diameter <0.1 μm may pass from the lungs into the systemic circulation.

The aim of this article is to provide an update on this subject, with particular emphasis on the link between PM and systemic hemostatic parameters. The authors discuss the physicochemical characteristics of PM, namely the size and composition as determinant factors in their effects, give a description of hemostasis by focusing on coagulation factors, platelets, and their role in thrombosis, and describe the state-of-the-art on this topic in relation to PM.

Physicochemical characteristics of particulate matter

PM consists of a wide range of solid or liquid particles. PM sizes range from 0.001 to 100 μm in aerodynamic diameter. The size distribution of particles in urban air is conventionally characterized by three modes [25]. The smallest of these sizes, <0.1 μm in diameter, is the nucleation mode and is formed by condensation of hot vapor from combustion sources and from chemical conversion of gases to particles in the atmosphere. Particles of this size have a high chance of deposition in the gas-exchanging (alveolar) part of the lung; they are relatively short-lived and grow into larger particles between 0.1 and approximately 1 μm in diameter, known as the accumulation mode. These particles remain suspended for up to several weeks in the air and are not readily removed by rain. The third size, the coarse mode, comprises particles larger than approximately 2 μm in diameter. These are generally formed by break-up of larger matter and include wind-blown dust and soil, particles from construction, and sea spray. Their size means that they remain in the air for relatively short periods, but they make (in relation to their numbers) a disproportionate contribution to PM_{10} mass when measured close to a source [25].

The size distribution used for regulation is slightly different and is defined as follows: $PM_{2.5}$ (fine particles) and PM_{10} refer to all particles with aerodynamic diameters <2.5 μm and 10 μm, respectively. They are measured according to the total mass of PM below the specified size per cubic meter of air. UFPs are measured according to the number of particles (counts) per cubic meter or centimeter of air because there are large numbers but small overall mass [26].

The epidemiologic and clinical studies have investigated mainly the link between PM_{10} or $PM_{2.5}$ and cardiovascular morbidity and mortality, but recent evidence (essentially from experimental studies) suggests that the ultrafine fraction of these particles shows more toxicity. These particles deposit in greater numbers and deeper into the lungs than larger particles. They also have a larger surface area than larger-sized particles, thus having greater potential for interactions with biologic targets and causing a greater inflammatory response [27,28]. UFPs are mainly emitted from combustion engines (eg, diesel-powered engines) and other high-temperature processes in the form of fractal-like aggregates composed of solid nanoparticles [29]. Because of the large increase in vehicle traffic, these UFPs are probably more frequent than in the past, when other sources of energy, such as coal or other fuels, were used. More than 100,000 particles per cm^3 may be found in the vicinity of a busy road [30].

The chemical composition of ambient airborne particles varies in time and space, depending on the activity of local and distant sources and meteorologic conditions [25]. Combustion processes produce particles based on carbon, carrying various metal compounds and organic chemicals derived from the fuel burnt. Photochemical reactions produce mainly ammonium sulfate and nitrate particles, derived in part from gases produced by combustion sources and in part from ammonia derived from animal sources. The proportion of these components varies in different seasons. In addition to this fine component, the coarser fraction may contain a wide variety of chemical substances, including salt, silicates, and biologic particles, depending on local sources [25].

Effect of particulate matter on hemostasis

In this section the authors describe the essential features of primary and secondary hemostasis and summarize and discuss the recent studies linking PM and hemostasis.

Hemostasis in physiologic and pathophysiologic conditions

Under physiologic conditions, hemostasis is finely balanced (ie, circulating blood contains procoagulant activity, counterbalanced by a compensatory damping effect by anticoagulant mechanisms). The coagulation is initiated within seconds after a blood vessel injury and occurs on the damaged endothelium. This process goes hand in hand with platelet-to-vessel wall adhesion, platelet-platelet interaction, and eventually hemostatic plug formation at the site of injury. This process is called primary hemostasis (Fig. 1). Secondary hemostasis essentially consists of coagulation triggered to form fibrin strands, which strengthen the platelet plug and arrest blood loss (Fig. 2). Activated platelets release the content of their granules, a process that amplifies primary hemostasis but also provides negatively charged phospholipids and coagulation cofactors.

The constituents of the hemostatic system

It should be pointed out that the endothelium, leukocytes, and erythrocytes all participate in the preservation of the integrity of the vasculature (see Fig. 1). The issue of acute PM interactions with inflammation and vascular endothelium is discussed in more detail in this issue in the article by Frampton. This article addresses PM effects on the coagulation cascade and platelets.

The coagulation cascade. In our current understanding, the process of clot formation is considered to be a two-stage process (ie, initiation of

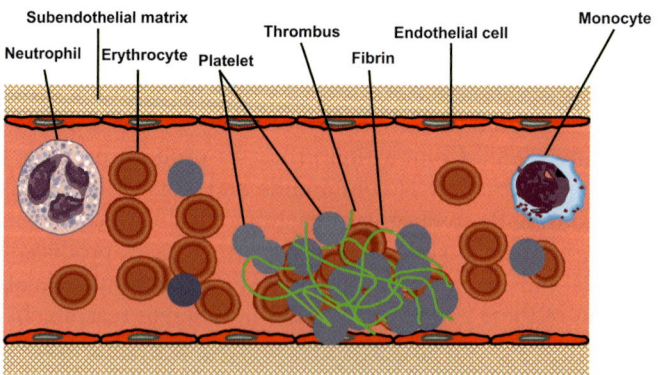

Fig. 1. Schematic representation of the constituents of the hemostatic system.

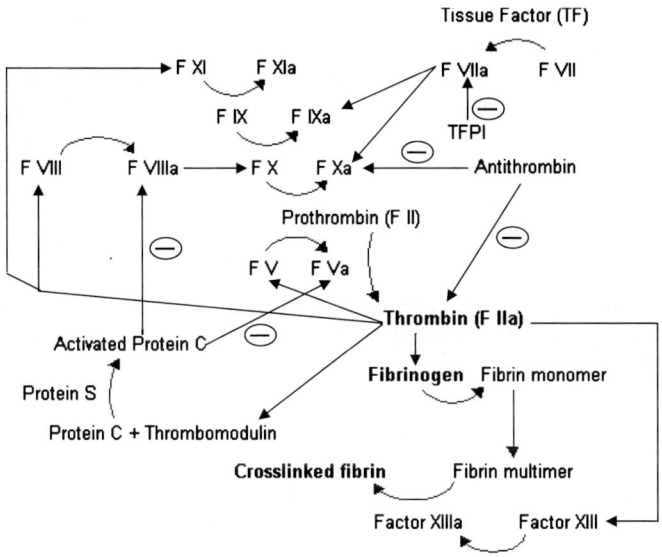

Fig. 2. Coagulation cascade and fibrin formation by TF. TFPI, tissue factor pathway inhibitor.

coagulation and propagation of the resultant thrombus). The initiation phase (see Fig. 2) begins when disruption of vessel walls exposes tissue factor (TF) to circulating Factor VII. TF forms a complex with Factor VIIa, which circulates in plasma in a higher amount than any other activated coagulation factor. After damage to the endothelium, TF is exposed and forms a complex with Factor VIIa (TF-FVIIa) upon binding to negatively charged surfaces. This occurrence activates Factor IX and Factor X. Factor VII itself is activated by thrombin, Factor XIa, plasmin, Factor XII, and Factor Xa. The activation of Factor Xa by TF-FVIIa is almost immediately inhibited by TF pathway inhibitor. Factor Xa and its co-factor Factor Va form the prothombinase complex, which activates prothrombin to the first traces of thrombin. Thrombin has a large array of functions. Its primary role is the conversion of fibrinogen to fibrin, the building block of a hemostatic plug. It also activates Factors VIII and V and their inhibitor protein C in the presence of thrombomodulin, and it activates Factor XIII, which forms covalent bonds that cross-link the fibrin polymers that form from activated monomers (see Fig. 2).

Platelets and thrombogenesis. The initiation of atherothrombosis involves a process of platelet adhesion, activation, and aggregation [31]. The initial event in the thrombotic process is the adhesion of platelets to the subendothelial matrix at the site of vascular damage. The platelet aggregate provides a surface for the assembly of procoagulant proteins. All coagulation factors must adhere to a surface to be optimally active. The platelet aggregate acts as a catalyst for the development of the thrombus and, ultimately, vessel occlusion when exacerbated.

During atherosclerosis, the disruption of an atherosclerotic plaque and exposure to elevated TF trigger a cascade of platelet-mediated events, which results in the formation of a platelet-rich thrombus at the site of injury [32].

Thrombosis can occur in veins or arteries. Venous thrombi, which form under low shear conditions, are predominantly composed of fibrin and red blood cells. The process can be triggered by direct injury to the vessel wall during surgery, after trauma, or by mechanical damage secondary to indwelling venous catheters. The thrombi can obstruct venous outflow and cause localized pain and swelling. The proximal venous thrombi are more likely to detach and embolize to the lung, a process that can be fatal [33]. Arterial thrombi form under high shear conditions and are comprised mainly of platelet aggregates held together by fibrin strands. Most arterial thrombi are superimposed on disrupted atherosclerotic plaques [32,34]. Rupture of the plaque exposes blood to thrombogenic material in the lipid-rich core. Platelets adhere to subendothelial collagen and von Willebrand factor, where they become activated and aggregate. Exposed TF triggers coagulation and induces the formation of fibrin strands that stabilize the platelet-rich thrombus. If the thrombus is of sufficient size to disrupt blood flow, shear increases and promotes additional platelet and fibrin deposition. Complete obstruction of arterial flow in coronary or cerebral vessels leads to irreversible ischemia, which manifests as a myocardial infarction or stroke, respectively [32,34]. Both have been consistently linked to PM (see later discussion) [19,20,35,36]. More specifically, platelets adhere to subendothelial matrix proteins, the two most important being collagen and von Willebrand factor [37,38]. These proteins interact with specific receptors on the surface of the platelet, collagen with glycoprotein VI and integrin $\alpha_2\beta_1$ and von Willebrand factor with the glycoprotein Ib/IX/V complex [39]. The result of these interactions is platelet adhesion and the formation of a monolayer of platelets. The interaction with these matrix proteins initiates platelet activation. Binding of these proteins to specific glycoproteins generates a molecular signal within the cell, which leads to activation of the fibrinogen receptor $\alpha_2\beta_3$ [40,41]. Platelet aggregation is accomplished by binding fibrinogen and other RGD (Arg-Gly-Asp)-containing adhesion ligands to the $\alpha_2\beta_3$ receptor. Platelets are also activated through other stimulatory platelet receptors for adenosine diphosphate, epinephrine, thrombin, and thromboxane A_2, among others [38].

Mechanistic studies linking particulate matter and coagulation and platelets

The mechanisms underlying the cardiovascular effects of particles are not fully understood. It has been suggested that inhaled particles may affect the autonomic nervous system, which can explain the PM effects on heart function, particularly rhythm [10,42]. Two other complementary hypotheses may explain the cardiovascular effects of PM. The first hypothesis is based on the occurrence of pulmonary inflammation, leading to the release of mediators, which may influence platelets, coagulation, or other cardiovascular endpoints [12,43]. The second hypothesis is that the particles translocate from the lungs into the systemic circulation and, directly or indirectly, influence hemostasis or cardiovascular integrity. The authors discuss these two hypotheses and their impact on coagulation and platelet function.

Systemic translocation as a potential mechanism for interaction between particulate matter and platelets and coagulation factors

Translocation of UFPs from the lungs into the systemic circulation is being increasingly investigated [24]. This issue is addressed in more detail in the article by Elder and Oberdörster elsewhere in this issue. Many years ago, Berry and colleagues [44] reported that ultrafine colloidal gold particles (30 nm) administered intratracheally in rats are able to translocate rapidly. The authors demonstrated the presence of particles in blood platelets of the alveolar capillaries within 30 minutes after their administration. The authors suggested that this translocation might have a double impact, the first being local, involving modification of the alveolo-capillary barrier by factors released by platelets, and the second impact being the delivery of potentially toxic material at distant sites. They also pointed out that phagocytosis of particles by platelets might predispose them to aggregation and thrombosis. Recently and in agreement with the findings of Berry and colleagues [44], the authors have shown that UFPs pass from the lungs into the blood circulation in hamsters [45]. In this study, they used 80 nm albumin-nanocolloid particles labeled radioactively with technetium-99 as a model of UFPs and studied their distribution in the blood and other organs after their intratracheal administration in the hamster. They demonstrated that a substantial fraction of ^{99m}Tc-albumin diffuses rapidly (within minutes and up to 1 hour) from the lungs into the systemic circulation [45]. In addition to our study performed in hamsters, others also have reported extrapulmonary translocation of UFPs after intratracheal instillation or inhalation to other animal species [46–48]. The amount of UFPs that translocated into blood and extrapulmonary organs differed among these studies, however. Research also has shown that after intranasal delivery, polystyrene microparticles (1.1 μm) can translocate to tissues in the systemic compartment [49]. Recent studies have provided morphologic data illustrating that inhaled particles are transported into the pulmonary capillary space, presumably by transcytosis [50,51].

In an ex vivo model of isolated perfused rat lungs, a preparation that lacks lymph flow and recruited inflammatory cells, Meiring and colleagues [52] have confirmed that UFPs can translocate from the lung into the circulation upon pharmacologic mediation (H_2O_2, vascular histamine administration), used to increase pulmonary microvascular permeability. Using

mast cells directly and increase histamine levels and symptom severity in humans [75,76]. The authors found that DEPs led to a significant prothrombotic tendency, activation of circulating blood platelets, and lung inflammation as early as 1 hour and persisting up to 24 hours. Pulmonary inflammation and peripheral thrombosis were correlated at 6 and 24 hours, but the prothrombotic tendency observed 1 hour after DEP exposure does not seem to correlate with pulmonary inflammation. The latter is compatible with direct platelet activation by DEP, having penetrated into the circulation [77]. In subsequent experiments, they found 24 hours after DEP exposure that pretreatment with dexamethasone, given intraperitoneally, intratracheally, or with cromoglycate, blocked DEP-induced pulmonary inflammation, prothrombotic events, and histamine release in BAL and plasma. They concluded that the systemic inflammatory and prothrombotic effects observed 24 hours after DEP administration are secondary to lung inflammation and that they can be prevented by mast cell stabilization [78].

It should be stressed that although the thrombosis model used normal healthy animals, it is a good model for the study of "compromised" individuals, such as thrombosis-prone patients. The authors did not investigate whether particles cause thrombosis but whether they can enhance peripheral vascular thrombosis when an endothelial lesion has been produced. This is a realistic experimental set-up for the human situation.

It is important to mention that in this study the authors measured soluble von Willebrand factor in plasma and recorded no effect after DEP administration compared with controls [78], although they found an enhancement of thrombosis. The findings are compatible with those of Gilmour and colleagues [79], who showed no increase of von Willebrand factor after exposure to fine or ultrafine carbon black particles in rats. Although these authors failed to show an increase of plasma fibrinogen, however [79], Gardner and colleagues [80] reported an increase in fibrinogen levels after exposure of rats to residual oil fly ash. This discrepancy can be explained by the nature of the particles instilled. Research has shown that fibrinogen levels were enhanced in pulmonary hypertensive rats instilled with diesel particles [81], which illustrates the need to study compromised animals that mimic humans with pre-existing cardiovascular diseases.

The authors have studied the relationship between pulmonary inflammation and thrombotic complications using the established model of sustained pulmonary inflammation induced by silica particles. They demonstrated that intratracheal instillation of silica particles leads to significant dose-dependent increases of macrophage and neutrophil numbers in BAL and the development of a prothrombotic tendency in circulating blood. By specifically depleting lung macrophages with clodronate-liposomes, they found that the influx of polymorphonuclear leukocyte in BAL and the peripheral thrombotic tendency were abrogated. The depletion of circulating neutrophils and monocytes by cyclophosphamide also abolished the cellular influx in BAL and the peripheral thrombotic tendency, despite normal numbers of

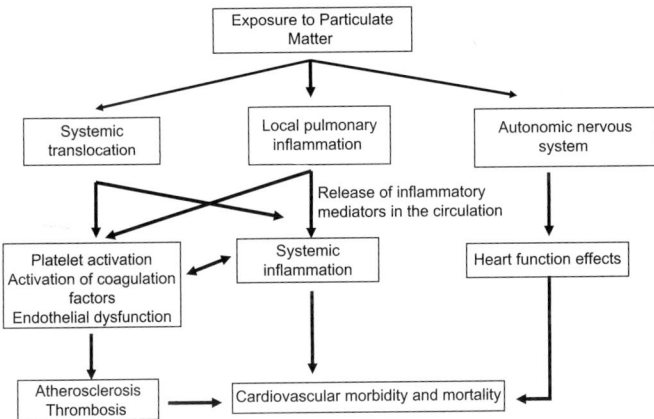

Fig. 4. Potential pathophysiologic mechanisms of particulate air pollution and cardiovascular effects.

lung macrophages. The authors found that silica caused an increase in neutrophil elastase activity in plasma. These findings uncover pulmonary macrophage-neutrophil cross-talk releasing neutrophil elastase into the blood circulation. Elastase, triggering activation of circulating platelets, may predispose platelets to initiate thrombotic events on mildly damaged vasculature.

With respect to atherosclerosis, two studies have assessed the possibility that the increased levels of circulating inflammatory mediators induced by PM cause progression and instability of atherosclerosis in Watanabe heritable hyperlipidemic rabbits that naturally develop atherosclerotic plaques [82,83]. These studies showed that 4 weeks of exposure of these animals to ambient particles induced a local inflammatory response in the lung, a systemic inflammatory response that included stimulation of the bone marrow, and caused progression of atherosclerosis in the aorta and coronary arteries [82,83].

Summary

There is strong evidence that particulate air pollution increases the risk of cardiovascular diseases. Fig. 4 summarizes some of the hypothesized pathways. In an effort to provide biologic plausibility for this association, several mechanistic studies have been performed, which have improved the understanding on how PM can affect platelets and the coagulation system and be responsible for the development of atherothrombosis complications. The authors still need to address several remaining questions: (1) What is the role of factors modulating particle translocation, such as the way of exposure, dose, size, surface chemistry, time course, and inflammatory mediators? (2) What are the mechanisms behind the cross-talk between lung macrophages, infiltrating granulocytes, mast cells, and the mediators involved in the activation of peripheral platelets and coagulation factors? (3) Which receptors present on blood platelets are responsible for the particle-induced platelet activation? (4) How do acute and chronic exposures and single versus repeated doses compare in healthy animals and animals with pre-existing cardiovascular diseases? (5) What are the critical chemical and biologic constituents of PM (eg, metals, carbon, polycyclic aromatic hydrocarbons, endotoxin) and what is the role of different PM size fractions, including UFPs (<0.1 μm) and the coarse fraction ($PM_{10 \text{ to } 2.5}$), in the adverse cardiovascular effects of air pollution?

References

[1] Samet JM, Dominici F, Curriero FC, et al. Fine particulate air pollution and mortality in 20 US cities, 1987–1994. N Engl J Med 2000;343:1742–9.

[2] Dockery DW, Schwartz J, Spengler JD. Air pollution and daily mortality: associations with particulates and acid aerosols. Environ Res 1992;59(2):362–73.

[3] Schwartz J. Air pollution and hospital admissions for cardiovascular disease in Tucson. Epidemiology 1997;8(4):371–7.

[4] Brunekreef B, Holgate ST. Air pollution and health. Lancet 2002;360(9341):1233–42.

[5] Schwartz J. Air pollution and daily mortality: a review and meta analysis. Environ Res 1994; 64(1):36–52.

[6] Wordley J, Walters S, Ayres JG. Short term variations in hospital admissions and mortality and particulate air pollution. Occup Environ Med 1997;54(2):108–16.

[7] Brook RD, Franklin B, Cascio W, et al. Air pollution and cardiovascular disease: a statement for healthcare professionals from the expert panel on population and prevention science of the American Heart Association. Circulation 2004;109(21):2655–71.

[8] Pope CA III, Verrier RL, Lovett EG, et al. Heart rate variability associated with particulate air pollution. Am Heart J 1999;138(5 Pt 1):890–9.

[9] Liao D, Creason J, Shy C, et al. Daily variation of particulate air pollution and poor cardiac autonomic control in the elderly. Environ Health Perspect 1999;107(7):521–5.

[10] Gold DR, Litonjua A, Schwartz J, et al. Ambient pollution and heart rate variability. Circulation 2000;101(11):1267–73.

[11] Peters A, Doring A, Wichmann HE, et al. Increased plasma viscosity during an air pollution episode: a link to mortality? Lancet 1997;349(9065):1582–7.

[12] Seaton A, Soutar A, Crawford V, et al. Particulate air pollution and the blood. Thorax 1999; 54(11):1027–32.

[13] Brook RD, Brook JR, Urch B, et al. Inhalation of fine particulate air pollution and ozone causes acute arterial vasoconstriction in healthy adults. Circulation 2002;105(13):1534–6.

[14] Peters A, Perz S, Doring A, et al. Increases in heart rate during an air pollution episode. Am J Epidemiol 1999;150(10):1094–8.

[15] Urch B, Silverman F, Corey P, et al. Acute blood pressure responses in healthy adults during controlled air pollution exposures. Environ Health Perspect 2005;113(8):1052–5.

[16] Schwartz J, Morris R. Air pollution and hospital admissions for cardiovascular disease in Detroit, Michigan. Am J Epidemiol 1995;142(1):23–35.

[17] Rich DQ, Schwartz J, Mittleman MA, et al. Association of short-term ambient air pollution concentrations and ventricular arrhythmias. Am J Epidemiol 2005;161(12):1123–32.

[18] Wellenius GA, Bateson TF, Mittleman MA, et al. Particulate air pollution and the rate of hospitalization for congestive heart failure among Medicare beneficiaries in Pittsburgh, Pennsylvania. Am J Epidemiol 2005;161(11):1030–6.

[19] Peters A, Dockery DW, Muller JE, et al. Increased particulate air pollution and the triggering of myocardial infarction. Circulation 2001;103(23):2810–5.

[20] Peters A, von Klot S, Heier M, et al. Exposure to traffic and the onset of myocardial infarction. N Engl J Med 2004;351(17):1721–30.

[21] Kunzli N, Jerrett M, Mack WJ, et al. Ambient air pollution and atherosclerosis in Los Angeles. Environ Health Perspect 2005;113(2):201–6.

[22] Nemmar A, Hoylaerts MF, Hoet PH, et al. Possible mechanisms of the cardiovascular effects of inhaled particles: systemic translocation and prothrombotic effects. Toxicol Lett 2004; 149(1–3):243–53.

[23] Utell MJ, Frampton MW, Zareba W, et al. Cardiovascular effects associated with air pollution: potential mechanisms and methods of testing. Inhal Toxicol 2002;14(12): 1231–47.

[24] Oberdorster G, Oberdorster E, Oberdorster J. Nanotoxicology: an emerging discipline evolving from studies of ultrafine particles. Environ Health Perspect 2005;113(7):823–39.

[25] Oberdorster G. Pulmonary effects of inhaled ultrafine particles. Int Arch Occup Environ Health 2001;74(1):1–8.

[26] Peters A, Wichmann HE, Tuch T, et al. Respiratory effects are associated with the number of ultrafine particles. Am J Respir Crit Care Med 1997;155(4):1376–83.

[27] Oberdorster G, Ferin J, Lehnert BE. Correlation between particle-size, in-vivo particle persistence, and lung injury. Environ Health Perspect 1994;102:173–9.

[28] Nemmar A, Delaunois A, Nemery B, et al. Inflammatory effect of intratracheal instillation of ultrafine particles in the rabbit: role of C-fiber and mast cells. Toxicol Appl Pharmacol 1999; 160(3):250–61.

[29] Xiong C, Friedlander SK. Morphological properties of atmospheric aerosol aggregates. Proc Natl Acad Sci U S A 2001;98(21):11851–6.

[30] Shi JP, Mark D, Harrison RM. Characterization of particles from a current technology heavy-duty diesel engine. Environ Sci Technol 2000;34:748–55.

[31] Melis E, Carmeliet P, Dewerchin M, et al. The importance of enzyme cofactors: tissue factor in blood coagulation and beyond. Recent Res Devel Biochem 2002;3(Part II):609–38.

[32] Libby P. Inflammation in atherosclerosis. Nature 2002;420(6917):868–74.

[33] Lensing AWA, Prandoni P, Prins MH, et al. Deep-vein thrombosis. Lancet 1999;353(9151): 479–85.

[34] Stone PH. Triggering myocardial infarction. N Engl J Med 2004;351(17):1716–8.

[35] Hong YC, Lee JT, Kim H, et al. Air pollution: a new risk factor in ischemic stroke mortality. Stroke 2002;33(9):2165–9.

[36] Hong YC, Lee JT, Kim H, et al. Effects of air pollutants on acute stroke mortality. Environ Health Perspect 2002;110(2):187–91.

[37] Chen JM, Lopez KA. Interactions of platelets with subendothelium and endothelium. Microcirculation 2005;12(3):235–46.

[38] Andrews RK, Gardiner EE, Shen Y, et al. Platelet interactions in thrombosis. IUBMB Life 2004;56(1):13–8.

[39] Zaffran Y, Meyer SC, Negrescu E, et al. Signaling across the platelet adhesion receptor glycoprotein Ib-IX induces alpha(IIb)beta(3) activation both in platelets and a transfected Chinese hamster ovary cell system. J Biol Chem 2000;275(22):16779–87.

[40] Nakamura T, Kambayashi J, Okuma M, et al. Activation of the GP IIb-IIIa complex induced by platelet adhesion to collagen is mediated by both alpha(2)beta(1) integrin and GP VI. J Biol Chem 1999;274(17):11897–903.

[41] Kuijpers MJE, Schulte V, Oury C, et al. Facilitating roles of murine platelet glycoprotein Ib and alpha IIb beta 3 in phosphatidylserine exposure during vWF-collagen-induced thrombus formation. J Physiol 2004;558(2):403–15.

[42] Riediker M, Cascio WE, Griggs TR, et al. Particulate matter exposure in cars is associated with cardiovascular effects in healthy young men. Am J Respir Crit Care Med 2004;169(8): 934–40.

[43] Seaton A, MacNee W, Donaldson K, et al. Particulate air pollution and acute health effects. Lancet 1995;345(8943):176–8.

[44] Berry JP, Arnoux B, Stanislas B, et al. A microanalytic study of particles transport across the alveoli: role of blood platelets. Biomedicine 1977;27:354–7.

[45] Nemmar A, Vanbilloen H, Hoylaerts MF, et al. Passage of intratracheally instilled ultrafine particles from the lung into the systemic circulation in hamster. Am J Respir Crit Care Med 2001;164(9):1665–8.

[46] Oberdorster G, Sharp Z, Atudorei V, et al. Extrapulmonary translocation of ultrafine carbon particle following whole-body inhalation exposure of rats. J Toxicol Environ Health A 2002;65(20):1531–43.

[47] Takenaka S, Karg E, Roth C, et al. Pulmonary and systemic distribution of inhaled ultrafine silver particles in rats. Environ Health Perspect 2001;109(Suppl 4):547–51.

[48] Kreyling W, Semmler M, Erbe F, et al. Translocation of ultrafine insoluble iridium particles from lung epithelium to extrapulmonary organs is size dependent but very low. J Toxicol Environ Health A 2002;65(20):1513–30.

[49] Eyles JE, Bramwell VW, Williamsson ED, et al. Microsphere translocation and immunopotentiation in systemic tissues following intranasal administration. Vaccine 2001;19(32):4732–42.

[50] Kato T, Yashiro T, Murata Y, et al. Evidence that exogenous substances can be phagocytized by alveolar epithelial cells and transported into blood capillaries. Cell Tissue Res 2003;311(1):47–51.

[51] Kapp N, Kreyling W, Schulz H, et al. Electron energy loss spectroscopy for analysis of inhaled ultrafine particles in rat lungs. Microsc Res Tech 2004;63(5):298–305.

[52] Meiring J, Borm PJA, Bagate K, et al. The influence of hydrogen peroxide and histamine on lung permeability and translocation of iridium nanoparticles in the isolated perfused rat lung. Part Fibre Toxicol 2005;2(3).

[53] Nemmar A, Hamoir J, Nemery B, et al. Evaluation of particle translocation across the alveolo-capillary barrier in isolated perfused rabbit lung model. Toxicology 2005;208(1):105–13.

[54] Nemmar A, Hoet PH, Vanquickenborne B, et al. Passage of inhaled particles into the blood circulation in humans. Circulation 2002;105:411–4.

[55] Simon BH, Ando HY, Gupta PK. Circulation time and body distribution of 14C-labeled amino-modified polystyrene nanoparticles in mice. J Pharm Sci 1995;84(10):1249–53.

[56] Kawakami K, Iwamura A, Goto E, et al. Kinetics and clinical application of 99mTc-technegas. Kaku Igaku 1990;27(7):725–33.

[57] Brown JS, Zeman KL, Bennett WD. Ultrafine particle deposition and clearance in the healthy and obstructed lung. Am J Respir Crit Care Med 2002;166(9):1240–7.

[58] Ghio AJ, Kim C, Devlin RB. Concentrated ambient air particles induce mild pulmonary inflammation in healthy human volunteers. Am J Respir Crit Care Med 2000;162(3 Pt 1):981–8.

[59] Huang YCT, Ghio AJ, Stonehuerner J, et al. The role of soluble components in ambient fine particles-induced changes in human lungs and blood. Inhal Toxicol 2003;15(4):327–42.

[60] Ghio AJ, Devlin RB. Inflammatory lung injury after bronchial instillation of air pollution particles. Am J Respir Crit Care Med 2001;164(4):704–8.

[61] van Eeden SF, Tan WC, Suwa T, et al. Cytokines involved in the systemic inflammatory response induced by exposure to particulate matter air pollutants (PM10). Am J Respir Crit Care Med 2001;164(5):826–30.

[62] Salvi S, Blomberg A, Rudell B, et al. Acute inflammatory responses in the airways and peripheral blood after short-term exposure to diesel exhaust in healthy human volunteers. Am J Respir Crit Care Med 1999;159(3):702–9.

[63] Blomberg A, Tornqvist H, Desmyter L, et al. Exposure to diesel exhaust nanoparticles does not induce blood hypercoagulability in an at-risk population. J Thromb Haemost 2005;3(9):2103–5.

[64] Kawasaki T, Kaida T, Arnout J, et al. A new animal model of thrombophilia confirms that high plasma factor VIII levels are thrombogenic. Thromb Haemost 1999;81(2): 306–11.

[65] Matsuno H, Uematsu T, Umemura K, et al. Effects of vapiprost, a novel thromboxane receptor antagonist, on thrombus formation and vascular patency after thrombolysis by tissue-type plasminogen activator. Br J Pharmacol 1992;106(3):533–8.

[66] Nemmar A, Hoylaerts MF, Hoet PHM, et al. Ultrafine particles affect experimental thrombosis in an *in vivo* hamster model. Am J Respir Crit Care Med 2002;166(7): 998–1004.

[67] Nemmar A, Hoylaerts M, Hoet PH, et al. Size effect of intratracheally instilled ultrafine particles on pulmonary inflammation and vascular thrombosis. Toxicol Appl Pharmacol 2003; 186:38–45.

[68] Silva VM, Corson N, Elder A, et al. The rat ear vein model for investigating in vivo thrombogenicity of ultrafine particles (UFP). Toxicol Sci 2005;85(2):983–9.

[69] Khandoga A, Stampfl A, Takenaka S, et al. Ultrafine particles exert prothrombotic but not inflammatory effects on the hepatic microcirculation in healthy mice in vivo. Circulation 2004;109(10):1320–5.

[70] Nemmar A, Hoet PH, Dinsdale D, et al. Diesel exhaust particles in lung acutely enhance experimental peripheral thrombosis. Circulation 2003;107(8):1202–8.

[71] Kundu SK, Heilmann EJ, Sio R, et al. Description of an in vitro platelet function analyzer–PFA-100. Semin Thromb Hemost 1995;21(Suppl 2):106–12.

[72] Zaca F, Benassi MS, Ghinelli M, et al. Myocardial infarction and histamine release. Agents Actions 1986;18(1–2):258–61.

[73] Clejan S, Japa S, Clemetson C, et al. Blood histamine is associated with coronary artery disease, cardiac events and severity of inflammation and atherosclerosis. J Cell Mol Med 2002; 6(4):583–92.

[74] Laine P, Kaartinen M, Penttila A, et al. Association between myocardial infarction and the mast cells in the adventitia of the infarct-related coronary artery. Circulation 1999;99(3): 361–9.

[75] Devouassoux G, Saxon A, Metcalfe DD, et al. Chemical constituents of diesel exhaust particles induce IL-4 production and histamine release by human basophils. J Allergy Clin Immunol 2002;109(5):847–53.

[76] Diaz-Sanchez D, Penichet-Garcia M, Saxon A. Diesel exhaust particles directly induce activated mast cells to degranulate and increase histamine levels and symptom severity. J Allergy Clin Immunol 2000;106(6):1140–6.

[77] Nemmar A, Nemery B, Hoet PHM, et al. Pulmonary inflammation and thrombogenicity caused by diesel particles in hamsters: role of histamine. Am J Respir Crit Care Med 2003; 168(11):1366–72.

[78] Nemmar A, Hoet PHM, Vermylen J, et al. Pharmacological stabilization of mast cells abrogates late thrombotic events induced by diesel exhaust particles in hamsters. Circulation 2004;110(12):1670–7.

[79] Gilmour PS, Ziesenis A, Morrison ER, et al. Pulmonary and systemic effects of short-term inhalation exposure to ultrafine carbon black particles. Toxicol Appl Pharmacol 2004; 195(1):35–44.

[80] Gardner SY, Lehmann JR, Costa DL. Oil fly ash-induced elevation of plasma fibrinogen levels in rats. Toxicol Sci 2000;56(1):175–80.

[81] Cassee FR, Boere AJF, Bos J, et al. Effects of diesel exhaust enriched concentrated PM2.5 in ozone preexposed or monocrotaline-treated rats. Inhal Toxicol 2002;14(7):721–43.

[82] Suwa T, Hogg JC, Quinlan KB, et al. Particulate air pollution induces progression of atherosclerosis. J Am Coll Cardiol 2002;39(6):935–42.

[83] Goto Y, Hogg JC, Shih CH, et al. Exposure to ambient particles accelerates monocyte release from bone marrow in atherosclerotic rabbits. Am J Physiol Lung Cell Mol Physiol 2004;287(1):L79–85.

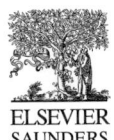

**ELSEVIER
SAUNDERS**

Clin Occup Environ Med
5 (4) 883–893

CLINICS IN
OCCUPATIONAL AND
ENVIRONMENTAL
MEDICINE

Implications for Occupational Exposure to Particulate Matter

Mark J. Utell, MD*, William S. Beckett, MD, MPH

*Medicine and Environmental Medicine, University of Rochester School of Medicine
and Dentistry, 575 Elmwood Avenue, Rochester, NY 14642, USA*

The recognition and study of respiratory system responses to particles encountered in the workplace has occurred over the past several centuries, initially stimulated by the recognition of premature death and illness in working groups exposed to specific particle substances and mixtures. Development of more sensitive measures of disease status, such as pulmonary function tests, and the evolution of epidemiologic, biostatistical, and computer analytical techniques has resulted in an expanded appreciation of the adverse effects of inhaled workplace particles on respiratory health. This recognition has led to establishment of limitations on exposures to workplace particles for specific substances in many countries. In most cases, ongoing research has led to a progressive lowering in the recommended limits for airborne concentrations of particles based on better understanding of the potential for adverse effects [1]. Limits for workplace particles are usually based on the assumption of exposures for intermittent work shifts (eg, five 8-hour work shifts over a 7-day period, with 16-hour periods without exposure between work days). The limits also assume exposure over an entire adult working life.

Epidemiologic studies that showed adverse effects of ambient air pollution particles on respiratory and general health beginning in 1960s and 1970s were not conceptually surprising [2]. The levels at which prolonged or constant exposures to particulate matter have been shown to affect acute and chronic health outcomes were surprising to many persons familiar with the levels of workplace dust, at which no apparent effect had been noted in long-term studies of working populations. Mechanisms for these effects of ambient particles were unknown. There are several possible explanations

---

* Corresponding author.
E-mail address: mark_utell@urmc.rochester.edu (M.J. Utell).

1526-0046/06/$ - see front matter © 2006 Elsevier Inc. All rights reserved.
doi:10.1016/j.coem.2006.07.001   *occmed.theclinics.com*

for the differences in the observed effects of ambient and occupational particles.

The first explanation may have to do with the different designs and capabilities of occupational dust versus ambient pollutant studies. Occupational studies most frequently take a group of working and exposed individuals and compare them with nonexposed controls, specifically with regard to lung disease outcomes. This design may omit study of individuals who have dropped out of the workforce because of disease and does not permit follow-up later in life for more delayed effects. Sample sizes are also usually limited by the number of workers in one or a limited group of workplaces, whereas air pollution studies can assess larger numbers of community members all exposed to the same ambient conditions and attain greater statistical power. The outcomes studied—lung diseases—also have been found not to be the most sensitive outcome measure for effects of prolonged exposures to ambient particles.

Another possible reason may be a "healthy worker effect," in which workplace exposures occur to adults with better-than-average health status, contrasted with community ambient air pollution studies, in which the excess mortality may occur in community members with lower levels of general health.

An additional difference between occupational and ambient exposures is the intermittent nature of occupational exposures, which might allow the respiratory and cardiovascular systems to recover from acute injury or clear particles in a manner not possible with constant or more prolonged ambient exposure.

A fourth possibility is that ambient particles, many of which are products of combustion, are more toxic on a mass concentration basis than the corresponding workplace particles associate with chronic lung disease. This possibility, which is currently under investigation in animal and human environmental exposure studies, would turn on its head the previous notion that industrial particles are invariably more toxic than ambient particles. It requires further investigation.

A corollary explanation may have to do with the presence of ultrafine particles in many ambient air pollution exposures. Ultrafine particles have a vastly greater total surface area than a comparable mass of fine particles. Because of their small size, they may enter the blood stream from the lungs more readily than larger particles. Because they tend to accumulate into larger particles rapidly when generated in high concentrations, ultrafine particles in the workplace might represent less of a health threat than ultrafine particles at lower concentrations in ambient air. Because of the difficulty in accurately measuring them, relatively little is known about exposures to ultrafine particles in the workplace.

Although each of these possible explanations might help to explain the rather striking differences between workplace exposures associated with disease and the much lower ambient particle levels, the apparent gap between occupational and ambient particle effects, based on current measures of mass concentrations dose-response effects, remains to be bridged scientifically.

Occupational particles and mechanisms of respiratory disease

The respiratory system has a limited repertoire of pathologic responses to inhaled substances. Occupational particles (including fibers) cause all the major categories of lung disease—rhinosinusitis, asthma, bronchitis, bronchiolitis, chronic obstructive pulmonary disease or emphysema, interstitial lung disease, pleural disease, cancer, and secondary pulmonary vascular disease (Table 1, Fig. 1). In the case of interstitial lung diseases caused by occupational particles, which are usually referred to as the inorganic dust pneumoconioses, particles of specific composition have been associated with specific lung diseases having a characteristic clinical picture and lung tissue histopathology (eg, coalworkers' pneumoconiosis, silicosis, asbestosis, chronic beryllium disease, hard metal pulmonary disease). More recently, many studies have shown that certain workplace particles are also associated with nonspecific lung diseases, such as chronic airflow obstruction and possibly nonspecific or "idiopathic" pulmonary fibrosis [3]. In many cases, the mechanisms by which particles cause the exposure-specific pneumoconioses are already much better understood than the mechanisms by which acute and chronic diseases are associated with ambient particles.

Historically, the definition of occupational lung disease has followed advances in medical science and technologic ability to describe diseases. In

Table 1
A selected listing of occupational respiratory diseases and the airborne particles that cause them

Disease	Causative particle/fiber
Rhinitis and laryngitis	Grain dusts (flours), latex coated corn-starch granules, pollens and mold spores, aerosolized metalworking fluids
Nasal ulceration and septal perforation	Arsenic, chromic acid, copper dust
Bronchitis	Rock and mineral dust, cement dust, silica
Bronchiolitis	Acetaldehyde
Asthma	Acid anhydrides, aldehydes, cobalt, flour and grain dust, ethylenediamine, latex
Chronic airflow obstruction	Coal dust, crystalline silica, cotton dust, cadmium
Pulmonary fibrosis	Asbestos, crystalline silica, kaolin, talc
Alveolar proteinosis	Crystalline silica, mixed dust
Hypersensitivity pneumonitis	Amebae, animal proteins, funal spores, trimellitic anhydride
Granulomatous disease	Beryllium
Inhalation fever	Cotton dust, freshly generated zinc oxide fumes, heated polytetraflouroethylene (Teflon)

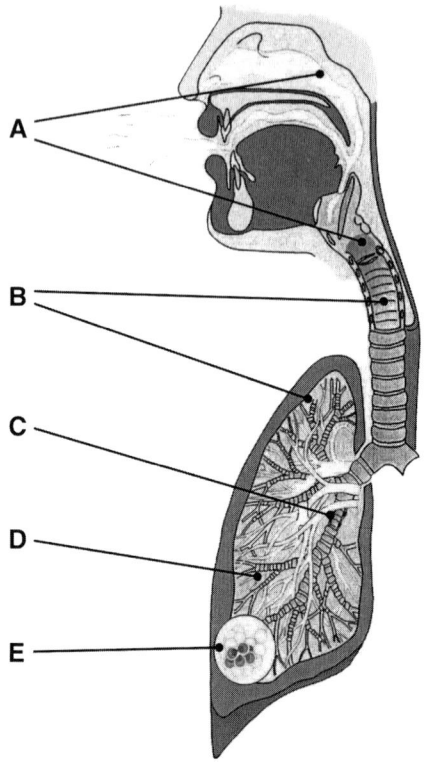

Fig. 1. Diagram of respiratory system, location of particle deposition by size, and types of occupational lung diseases by anatomic location. (*A*) Rhinitis and laryngitis. Largest particles impact in nose, pharynx, and larynx. More soluble gases (eg, sulfur dioxide) are absorbed by upper respiratory mucous membranes and cause edema and mucus hypersecretion. (*B*) Tracheitis, bronchitis, and bronchiolitis. Large particles (>10 μm aerodynamic diameter) are deposited and cleared by cilia. Smaller particles and fine fibers are deposited in bronchioles and bifurcations of alveolar ducts. (*C*) Asthma and chronic obstructive pulmonary disease. Allergens and irritants deposited on large airways by turbulent flow cause chronic inflammatory changes. (*D*) Cancer. Carcinogens (eg, asbestos, polycyclic aromatic hydrocarbons) contact bronchial epithelial cells and cause mutations in proto-oncogenes and tumor suppressor genes. Multiple hits result in malignant transformation. (*E*) Interstitial and pleural disease. Smallest particles (<10 μm diameter) and fibers are deposited in terminal bronchioles, alveolar ducts, and alveoli. Penetration to interstitium results in fibrosis and granuloma formation.

renaissance Europe, occupational lung disease was defined by a patient's symptoms, physical findings, and premature disability, as in "miners' pthisis" described by Agricola in the sixteenth century [4]. Widespread adoption of chest radiography in the early twentieth century introduced new radiographic patterns of pneumoconiosis [5]. Systematic collections of lung pathology from autopsies were uncommon at that time, and the surgical techniques that safely permitted open lung biopsy became widely used only in the second half of the twentieth century. This development permitted the association of a specific workplace exposure with a specific pulmonary histopathology, as in coalworkers' pneumoconiosis, welders' siderosis, silicosis, asbestosis, chronic beryllium lung disease, and hard metal pulmonary disease. A further refinement—the epidemiologic application of spirometry as a test of lung function—also was applied until the second half of the twentieth century. Finally, refinements in biostatistical techniques made epidemiologic analysis more sensitive to smaller adverse effects of exposure, and the application of computer technology to epidemiology made possible the multivariable analytic techniques to large databases that would have been prohibitively complex using simpler calculating machines.

Based on patterns of exposure, occupational lung diseases caused by particles are divided into inorganic dust pneumoconiosis, caused by mineral and metal dusts, and the organic dust diseases—primarily, hypersensitivity pneumonitis caused by micro-organisms and other biologic materials. Characteristics of inhaled particles that are associated with lung disease incidence or severity include not only the chemical composition of the particles but also particle size, freshness of generation of freshly cleaved crystalline particles (in the case of silicosis), exposure in combination with other metals (as in the case of cobalt and tungsten carbide), and the intensity of exposure (as in the case of silicoproteinosis) [6].

Although particles and fibers may contribute to all the major categories of respiratory system diseases, we have selected several examples of chronic dust diseases of the lung parenchyma, or pneumoconioses, for discussion.

Iron oxide and welders' siderosis

Iron oxide dust inhaled into the lungs of welders and metal polishers using iron oxide rubbing compounds can produce a chest radiographic picture of pneumoconiosis that is similar to relatively mild silicosis. Pulmonary function surveys did not find an association with lung function loss, and autopsy study of welders who died from other causes found that the deposits of iron oxide were not associated with fibrosis. The radiographic changes were found to clear when welders were followed up [7]. Welders' siderosis is an example of a "benign pneumoconiosis" in which dust deposition is radiographically visible but has little effect on lung function or health status.

Silica and silicosis

By contrast, freshly generated respirable crystalline silicon dioxide (silica) particles have a marked injurious effect on the respiratory system. Intense acute exposures can cause accelerated silicosis or silicoproteinosis, leading to death of otherwise healthy adults within months to a few years of exposure. Chronic exposure can lead to chronic bronchitis, chronic airflow obstruction, a severe and progressive pneumoconiosis, and premature mortality [8]. The presence of pneumoconiosis is also associated with increased risk for lung cancer [9]. Serious adverse effects of silica on the respiratory system are related at least in part to their ability to stimulate generation of reactive oxygen species by lung cells, possibly through the induction of tumor necrosis factor-alpha, and with a subsequent inflammatory response mediated by cytokines from cells activated in this process [10,11]. Silica is a mineral for which inter-individual variation in susceptibility is relatively unimportant compared with some other minerals, because with sufficient exposure most individuals develop the disease. As a common, naturally occurring mineral, silica exposures occur with inhalation of windblown crustal particles, although this occurrence has been shown to be clinically significant only under unusual conditions for humans and domesticated animals. The generation of high levels of freshly fractured, small particles through the use of powered mining or construction equipment and the generation of high levels of dust in workplace environments are most often associated with lung disease.

Asbestos (fiber) and asbestosis

The generic term "asbestos" is used to describe a group of commercially useful hydrated magnesium silicate minerals that, when crushed, break into fibers rather than dust. These inhaled fibers can cause a spectrum of disease, including malignancies and disorders of inflammation and fibrosis. Nonmalignant conditions include pleural plaques, pleural effusions, diffuse pleural thickening, asbestosis, and occasionally airflow obstruction. The major malignancies linked with asbestos exposure are carcinoma of the lung and diffuse malignant mesothelioma.

Despite the many years of investigation into asbestos-related disease, important controversies and uncertainties remain, including criteria for attributing lung cancer to asbestos exposure, radiographic criteria for diagnosing asbestos, relative toxicity of the various fiber types, and clinical significance of pleural plaques.

Asbestosis is a form of diffuse interstitial pulmonary fibrosis that results from the inhalation and deposition of large numbers of asbestos fibers, usually as a consequence of prolonged and repeated exposures. Classically, a patient with asbestosis experiences dyspnea, demonstrates rales on physical examination, has restrictive-type physiology on lung function testing, and has a chest radiograph that shows irregular opacities, predominantly in the lower lung fields with diffuse parenchymal fibrosis and associated pleural plaques. Chronic airflow obstruction has been described in asbestosis in persons who never smoked, but this is relatively uncommon [12]. A history of working in an asbestos industry and a latency of some 20 years or more since initial exposure are important features in establishing a diagnosis.

Fiber analyses of lung tissue in asbestosis reveal high lung burdens, two to three orders of magnitude greater than fiber burdens detected in occupationally unexposed controls, and the burdens increase with intensity of fibrosis. Most inhaled fibers deposit in the upper airways and at bifurcations, and few fibers that enter the trachea penetrate to the alveoli to be retained in the interstitium. Deposition, dissolution, and clearance of fibers vary considerably between chrysotile (serpentine) asbestos and the different amphibole (straight and needle-like) fibers. Chrysotile is less able to penetrate the deep lung because of its aerodynamic characteristics and is considerably more soluble; the half-lives of chrysotile versus amphiboles are of the order of months and years, respectively [13]. The deposited fibers stimulate macrophages to produce mediators and attract neutrophils. Oxygen radicals also contribute to tissue injury. Ultimately, fibroblast proliferation results and collagen production occurs.

There continues to be some debate regarding the radiographic criteria for diagnosing asbestosis. The profusion of small linear opacities on chest radiographs caused by lung fibrosis can be graded on a scale of 0 to 3 using the ILO International Classification of Radiographs of Pneumoconioses. For example, an American Thoracic Society committee in 1986 concluded that chest roentgenographic evidence of small irregular opacifications of a profusion of 1/1 or more was required to diagnose asbestosis [14], whereas the 2004 ATS committee concluded that profusion 1/0 was adequate. Whether asbestosis is a prerequisite for attributing lung cancer to asbestos exposure remains controversial. The interpretation of the data provides a wide range of opinions on criteria for attribution of lung cancer to asbestos, ranging from (1) a requirement for underlying radiographic asbestosis to (2) an increased quantitative fiber burden count in lung tissue even in the absence of asbestosis to (3) the presence of a history of asbestos exposure in the absence of other radiographic findings useful in documenting exposure.

The pleural plaque is recognized as a specific marker of fiber exposure, although the mechanism of plaque formation is not clear. The combination of discrete pleural plaques and interstitial fibrosis is highly diagnostic for asbestosis and virtually eliminates the need for more invasive diagnostic approaches. Plaques per se have little, if any, effect on pulmonary function in contrast to diffuse pleural thickening, which can result in significant decrements in lung function. Compared with individuals who do not have plaques, the presence of asbestos plaques is associated with an increased risk of mesothelioma. This presence presumably reflects increased exposure, however, because there is no evidence that plaques degenerate or evolve into malignancies [12]. The standard plain chest radiograph is an appropriate method for imaging of plaques; the use of high-resolution CT, although more sensitive, should be restricted to selected questions regarding evaluation of questionable pleural abnormalities.

Regulatory strategies have been enacted such that the current standards virtually eliminate the risk of asbestosis, assuming there is compliance with the workplace limits. Within public buildings and schools, the ambient levels are usually low and there should be no risk of asbestosis. It should be recognized, however, that the standards that are protective against asbestosis do not protect against mesothelioma, an uncommon but highly malignant tumor.

Chronic beryllium disease

The metallic element beryllium can cause acute inhalation pneumonitis and chronic disease that involves lung, lymph nodes, skin, and liver. Either the acute or the chronic form of the disease may be fatal. Chronic beryllium disease that involves the respiratory system is a granulomatous disease that commonly involves lung parenchyma and lymph nodes. A minority of individuals industrially exposed seem to develop disease, and disease may be absent in some persons with higher exposures, although it may be present in some individuals with lower exposures. Chronic beryllium disease seems to be a particle-induced disease for which a gene by environmental interaction is important in determining which exposed individuals will develop sensitization to the metal, a precursor of disease. The presence of a glutamic acid at residue 69 in the human leukocyte antigen-DPB1 gene (Glu69) is associated with increased risk for chronic beryllium disease [15].

Chronic beryllium disease also has been described in residents of a neighborhood close to a beryllium manufacturing plant, which indicates that beryllium dust also may be an "air toxic" pollutant [16].

Organic particles: hypersensitivity pneumonitis

In contrast to the inhalation of fibers, inorganic dusts, or most metals, inhaled organic antigens produce a parenchymal reaction of the lung in sensitized individuals, so-called "hypersensitivity pneumonitis." The individual becomes sensitized over time from repeated exposures, and disease requires the immunologically primed host and repeated exposures. The most common occupational antigens are proteins derived from bacteria, fungi, and animal species; less frequently, inhaled reactive chemicals can act as haptens and become antigenic when bound to the host's proteins [17].

In hypersensitivity pneumonitis, diagnostic approaches often include bronchoscopy with bronchoalveolar lavage. The characteristic findings include an alveolar lymphocytosis predominantly of the T-suppressor subtype (CD8+), and the CD4+ /CD8+ ratio is usually increased in the hours after exposure. Poorly formed granulomas can be seen on biopsy. High-resolution CT imaging is usually abnormal and shows patchy ground glass alveolar infiltrates. Antigen-specific immunoglobulin G antibodies are often present in the serum and lavage fluid. When precipitins are negative, as occurs in approximately one third of presumed cases of farmer's lung, it seems likely that testing was performed with the wrong antigen.

Hypersensitivity pneumonitis can present as an acute febrile illness, a subacute process characterized by progressive dyspnea, or a chronic irreversible process manifested most frequently as parenchymal fibrosis. Occasionally, however, it presents as emphysema as a consequence of farmer's lung [18]. During the acute episode, the individual appears ill and demonstrates inspiratory rales; recovery usually ensues with no residual damage.

Why an individual develops the acute, subacute, or chronic form of hypersensitivity pneumonitis raises interesting questions and remains under investigation. As with inorganic particles, dosimetry—including duration of exposure and particle concentration—is important. Finally, unique antigenic properties may lead to different disease presentations.

In contrast to the workplace standards for inorganic particles, there are currently few workplace standards for organic antigenic substances, and surveillance of antigen exposure by monitoring particle levels may not be adequate for preventing disease. The level of antigen may not be correlated with the total particle load. Once sensitized to an antigen, a worker may experience acute symptoms with low-level exposures to offending organic agents or chemicals, such as toluene diisocyanate.

Particles containing endotoxin: byssinosis

The term "byssinosis" is applied to acute and chronic diseases of the airways that occur in persons exposed to three vegetable fibers: cotton, flax (which is woven into linen), and soft hemp (which is used for making rope and net) [19]. Byssinosis includes the acute syndrome of chest tightness, dyspnea, and reversible airway obstruction that occurs at work within a few hours of exposure to cotton dust and the more severe and chronic disease, in which chest tightness and dyspnea may be present each day at work and eventually at all times. Organic dust toxic syndrome, a delayed febrile response to these dusts, may occur after inhalation of various organic materials that have been kept in conditions that permit the profuse growth of contaminating micro-organisms.

Worldwide, many more workers are exposed to cotton dust than to hemp or jute. Cotton is a plant-derived cellulose fiber. The long, thin, flexible cotton fiber consists of glucose units connected by glycosidic linkages that contain reactive hydrogen groups. Disease is largely the result of inhalation of the dust of the bract (dry, friable materials at the base of the cotton flower), leaf, and stem of the cotton plant, however.

Byssinosis is a nonallergic airways disease. In contrast to hypersensitivity pneumonitis, bronchoconstriction can be induced in previously unexposed persons with a first challenge to cotton dust. Although the mechanisms of and the etiologic agents that cause byssinosis remain incompletely understood, the acute response of byssinosis correlates better with the measured exposure to endotoxin (from the cell walls of contaminating gram-negative bacteria), whereas chronic air flow obstruction correlates better with total dust exposure. There are several other industries in which exposure to organic dusts heavily contaminated with endotoxin occurs, and symptoms of byssinosis are rarely reported. A distinct inflammatory airways response to contaminated bacterial endotoxin, other bacteria-derived substances, or other components of cotton dust has been linked to the chronic bronchitis associated with long-term exposure to cotton dust.

Reduction in total exposure to cotton dust is the primary treatment of byssinosis and is effective in preventing onset of disease and recurrence. Reduction can be achieved by controlling airborne dust levels with improved ventilation and prewashing of the cotton dust. The Occupational Safety and Health Administration cotton dust standard has been generally protective in preventing disease.

Summary

The demonstrated effects of lower levels of ambient particles on cardiovascular and respiratory system morbidity and mortality, summarized in detail in the first eight articles in this issue, were initially surprising in light of current concepts of occupational particle exposure and acute and chronic cardiopulmonary effects. Specifically, the exposure levels, as defined by the weight of particles per liter of breathing air, at which recognized disease occurs under workplace conditions are considerably higher than the observed levels of ambient particles associated with serious adverse health effects. The possible reasons for this difference have not been adequately addressed. To further address this question, a re-examination of workplace exposure response relationships is needed, which may include emphasis on measuring exposures to fine and ultrafine particles rather than to total particle mass concentration alone.

References

[1] American Conference of Governmental Industrial Hygienists. Documentation of the TLVs and BEIs. Cincinnati (OH): American Conference of Governmental Industrial Hygienists; 2005.

[2] Lave LB, Seskin EP. The relationship between daily mortality and daily air pollution. In: Lave LB, Seskin EP, editors. Air pollution and human health. Baltimore (MD): John Hopkins University Press; 1977. p. 186–209.

[3] Baumgartner KB, Samet JM, Coultas DB, et al. Occupational and environmental risk factors for idiopathic pulmonary fibrosis: a multicenter case-control study. Am J Epidemiol 2000;152:307–15.

[4] Agricola G, De re metallica. [Translated from the first Latin edition of 1556, with biographical introduction, annotations, and appendices upon the development of mining methods, metallurgical processes, geology, mineralogy & mining law from the earliest times to the 16th century.]. New York: Dover Publications; 1950.

[5] Pancoast HK, Pendergrass EP. Pneumoconiosis: a roentgenological study with notes on pathology. New York: Paul B. Hoeber, Inc; 1926.

[6] Oberdörster G, Driscoll KE, editors. Toxicology of natural and man-made fibrous and non-fibrous particles. Environ Health Perspect 1997;105(Suppl 5):1001–380.

[7] Doig AT, McLaughlin ATG. Clearing of x-ray shadows in welders. Lancet 1948;1:786–91.
[8] Ziskind M, Jones RN, Weill H. Silicosis: state of the art. Am Rev Respir Dis 1976;113: 643–65.
[9] American Thoracic Society. Adverse effects of crystalline silica exposure. Am J Respir Crit Care Med 1997;155:761–5.
[10] Vallyathan V, Shi X, Castranova V. Reactive oxygen species: their relation to pneumoconiosis and carcinogenesis. Environ Health Perspect 1998;106(Suppl 5):1151–5.
[11] Barrett EG, Johnston C, Oberdörster G, et al. Silica-induced chemokine expression in alveolar type II cells is mediated by TNF-α. Am J Physiol 1999;276:L979–88.
[12] American Thoracic Society. Diagnosis and initial management of nonmalignant diseases related to asbestos. Am J Respir Crit Care Med 2004;170:691–715.
[13] De Vuyst P, Gevenois PA. Asbestosis. In: Hendricks DJ, Burge PS, Beckett WS, et al, editors. Occupational disorders of the lung. Philadelphia: WB Saunders; 2002. p. 143–62.
[14] American Thoracic Society. The diagnosis of nonmalignant diseases related to asbestos. Am Rev Respir Dis 1986;134:363–8.
[15] Maier L, Martyny J, Mroz M, et al. Genetic and environmental risk factors in beryllium sensitization and chronic beryllium disease. Chest 2002;121(3 Suppl):81S.
[16] Eisenbud M, Wanta RC, Dustan C, et al. Non-occupational berylliosis. J Ind Hyg Toxicol 1949;31:282–94.
[17] Cormier Y. Hypersensitivity pneumonitis. In: Hendricks DJ, Burge PS, Beckett WS, et al, editors. Occupational disorders of the lung. Philadelphia: WB Saunders; 2002. p. 229–40.
[18] Erkinjuntti-Pekkanen R, Rythonen H, Kokkarinen JI, et al. Long-term outcome of farmer's lung evaluated by high resolution computed tomography: a case-control study. Am J Respir Crit Care Med 1998;158:662–5.
[19] Beckett WS, Utell MJ. Byssinosis and respiratory disease caused by vegetable dusts. In: Baum GL, Crapo JD, Celli BR, et al, editors. Textbook of pulmonary diseases. 6th edition. Philadelphia: Lippincott-Raven; 1998. p. 721–5.

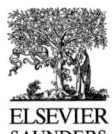

ELSEVIER
SAUNDERS

Clin Occup Environ Med
5 (4) 895–898

CLINICS IN
OCCUPATIONAL AND
ENVIRONMENTAL
MEDICINE

Index

Note: Page numbers of article titles are in **boldface** type.

1526-0046/06/$ - see front matter © 2006 Elsevier Inc. All rights reserved.
doi:10.1016/S1526-0046(06)00074-4   *occmed.theclinics.com*

Moving?

Make sure your subscription moves with you!

To notify us of your new address, find your **Clinics Account Number** (located on your mailing label above your name), and contact customer service at:

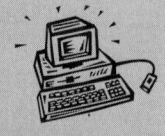

E-mail: elspcs@elsevier.com

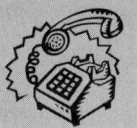

800-654-2452 (subscribers in the U.S. & Canada)
407-345-4000 (subscribers outside of the U.S. & Canada)

Fax number: 407-363-9661

Elsevier Periodicals Customer Service
6277 Sea Harbor Drive
Orlando, FL 32887-4800

*To ensure uninterrupted delivery of your subscription, please notify us at least 4 weeks in advance of move.

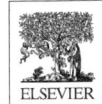
ELSEVIER